Garlic

Nature's Perfect Prescription

By
C. Gary Hullquist, M.D.

TEACH Services, Inc.
Brushton, New York

Published by

TEACH Services, Inc.
Route 1, Box 182
Brushton, New York 12916

CONTENTS

Perfect Prescription

Our apothecary's shop is our garden full of pot-herbs;
our doctor is a clove of garlic.
                              anonymous, 1615.

"Consider the lilies," the Great Teacher once said.

Garlic is certainly worth considering. *Allium sativum,* best known for its edible aromatic bulb, is a member of the lily family along with onions, shallots, leeks and chives. This compound bulb composed of individual "cloves" has been a favorite food and medicine for at least 4,000 years and probably longer.

Not surprisingly, this herb of the ancients has accumulated a vast heritage of both superstitious and scientific distinction. On one hand garlic was esteemed for its magical-mystical powers, and widely used as a protecting charm against vampires, werewolves and other evil forces. But at the same time, an impressive number of historical and anecdotal accounts were building garlic's reputation as a useful therapeutic food.

Garlic's ability to treat infections, reduce blood pressure, cure cancer and an amazing array of additional human maladies is now creating considerable interest among today's medical community and has catapulted this cloven aromatic bulb from the realm of culinary folklore to academic stardom.

Herbologist, Edward E. Shook complemented garlic with the following eulogy:

*"This lily is one of nature's great masterpieces
as a safe and certain remedy
for many of man's serious and devastating diseases."*

Today, the ancient Egyptian medical references to this masterpiece of nature are joined by well over a thousand scientific papers reporting the amazing medicinal merits of the pungent vegetable. A landmark comprehensive review of the literature was published in 1985 over three issues of *Critical Reviews in Food Science and Nutrition.* That same year Professor of Chemistry at New York State University at Albany, Eric Block, published *The Chemistry of Garlic and Onions* and captured the attention of both the scientific and general world. See *Scientific American* (252) 114–119, 1985.

But the practical application of garlic's many physiological virtues has been mostly limited to the purveyors of alternative medicine—health food stores, naturopaths, and vitamin enthusiasts. Mainstream medicine has been particularly slow in adopting nonprescription therapies, even those with documented and proven efficacy. There are understandable reasons for this behavior.

Competing theories in medicine operate under alternative paradigms (different points of view) and influence the way we look at and process new information. When one suggests that a particular *food* has medicinal value, skepticism is a natural response (within the pharmaceutical paradigm of medical therapeutics). And the lack of investigative initiative on the part of the pharmaceutical industry is likewise completely expected.

Medical research is extremely expensive. And why dump precious funds into the research of a naturally occurring pharmacological substance when it can't be patented? It's just not cost-effective. But the empirical evidence can no longer be ignored. A vast collection of recent technical publications is providing more than sufficient reason for many leading medical research facilities, hospitals and medical centers to make a new and serious reappraisal of **Nature's Perfect Prescription.**

Pharmacological Effects

Wow! Just look at what you can do with this gifted clove:

Garlic Decreases	Garlic Increases
Bacteria, yeast, fungi counts	
Cholesterol levels, synthesis, storage	Cholesterol elimination
Triglycerides levels	Triglyceride elimination
LDL and VLDL	HDL
Human gastric lipase levels	
Total liver lipids	Lipid excretion
Plasma fibrinogen	Fibrinolytic activity
Platelet aggregation & clotting	Blood coagulation time
Blood pressure	Blood vessel dilation
Blood sugar levels	Blood insulin levels
Prostaglandin production	Anti-inflammatory response
Free radicals	Glutathione peroxidase levels
Radiation toxicity	Radiation tolerance
Heavy metal toxicity	Heavy metal excretion rates
Nitrosamine production	Heavy metal binding capacity
Risk of gastric cancer	Anti-leukemic lymphocytes

Medline, the nation's largest medical research computer database, includes hundreds of citations reporting the effectiveness of garlic in

- killing bacteria, yeasts, fungi and viruses
- lowering cholesterol levels
- lowering high blood pressure
- preventing blood clots
- reducing the risk of stroke and heart attacks

- increasing immunity and disease resistance
- preventing cancer and its spread

The Lily of Legend

Chefs have often called it a 'stinking rose', but garlic is actually a variety of onion with a bulb sporting from four to fifteen cloves. There are three important varieties: American (Creole), Italian, and Tahiti. The American has a white skin and has the strongest flavor. The Italian has the most cloves and a pink skin. The Tahiti variety is the largest and measures up to three inches across.

The name originates from two old Anglo-Saxon words: *gar* (a spear) and *lac* (a plant) and refers to the shape of its leaves. Garlic has been used by cooks for centuries to turn the taste buds in diners of Italian spaghetti sauce, Chinese dishes, Middle Eastern hummus and hundreds of other famous foods because of its unique flavor.

No discussion of garlic would be complete without bringing up the subject of 'Garlic Breath.' Some have identified the responsible compound as a metabolic by-product of allicin called allymercaptan. It diffuses out of the blood stream during its circulation through the pulmonary vessels and during exhalation can flavor enhance your ambience.

Of course, as is often advised, the proper maximum dose of garlic can be easily determined by simply increasing the amount you consume each day until you start to notice people backing away from you when you approach.

We offer this advice 'clove in cheek.' But one serious piece of anecdotal trivia comes from a long time (5 year) dedicated garlic enthusiast who says he uses it daily, fresh and "lots of it"—at least 2 cloves a day. He, too, experienced the odor of garlic wafting on his breath and seeping from his skin that all initiates notice. But he claims it lasted only for the first few weeks. His interpretation of this encouraging phenomena is that his body "kicked garbage or toxins out" of his system.

But in addition to its reputation as a strong-scented seasoning, garlic is today becoming even more appreciated for its potential as a healing food. This is not actually late breaking news. The medicinal benefits of garlic and other bulbs of its ilk were common knowledge hundreds of years ago. One anonymous wit captured the essence of its medicinal talents in the following couplet:

> *"Eat onions in March and garlic in May*
> *Then the rest of the year, your doctor can play."*

In spite of such rational thought, superstition abounded. Appalachian asafetida, amulets of parsley worn around the neck, date back to medieval practices of wearing and displaying garlic strings as a means of securing supernatural protection. For example, Odysseus in ancient Greece saved himself from being rudely morphed into a pig by clutching a garlic clove. Now *that's* superstition.

Fortunately, there were plenty of other observers who recorded the benefits of *eating* rather than simply touching this magical herb.

Egyptian slaves working on the pyramid project depended on garlic's legendary ability to boost energy, strength and endurance. An inscription in the great Cheops states that 100,000 men were employed on its construction and "these ate garlic, leeks, and onions to the value of 1,600 talents of silver" (a cool million or two greenbacks at today's market value).

When the children of Israel, who slaved to build the pyramids, were later journeying in the wilderness after their exodus from Egypt, they fondly remembered "the leeks, and the onions, and the garlick...which we did eat in Egypt freely." Numbers 11:5 (the only reference in all Scripture to garlic). Meanwhile, back in Pharaoh's court references to garlic in the popular medical journals of the day indicate that it was employed to treat a list of some 22 ailments ranging from heart conditions to tumors.

Garlic's status as the Lily of the Nile ranked so high that the Roman poet Virgil pegged it as an Egyptian deity and noted that its consumption was prohibited by any of the priestly caste. While the Romans didn't imbibe in garlic worship they esteemed the noble bulb as 'the herb of Mars' and ceremoniously feasted on garlic in honor of the war god as they prepared for battle.

The Roman Medical Association expanded garlic's medicinal applications to include over 60 disorders including ulcers, asthma, and rheumatism. Pliny, the Roman historian, boasted that it had "very powerful properties" including its ability to drive away serpents and scorpions...friends and neighbors.

Long before Roman times, Hippocrates in ancient Greece classified garlic as an effective laxative and diuretic. No doubt he was thinking of garlic when he advised his fellow physicians: "Let food be your medicine." He also recognized the topical application of garlic by prescribing it as a steam fumigation for the treatment of uterine cancer.

Other Greeks of import, like Aristotle, Dioscorides, and Sotion, also sang its praises.

Galen listed garlic as a general antidote for poisons and eulogized the plant as a "theriac" or panacea for all diseases. Mohammed shared the opinion concerning garlic's capacity as an antidote and observed that when garlic is "applied on the sting of a scorpion or the bite of the viper it produces favorable results."

Vikings and Phoenicians carried large quantities of garlic on their long ocean voyages. Legendary Dr. Albert Schweitzer used garlic for treating typhoid fever and cholera. And East Indian, Chinese and Japanese practitioners continue to use garlic for lowering blood pressure and preventing atherosclerotic heart disease.

Its long romantic history and its remarkable curative virtues wrap this oldest medicinal remedy in both respect and mystique.

Active Ingredients

A single garlic clove weighs in at just four calories but packs an impressive array of important minerals including

- **potassium**
- **calcium**
- **iron**
- **magnesium**
- **phosphorus**
- **zinc**
- **copper**
- **sulfur**
- **germanium**
- **selenium**

and the B vitamin, **thiamine**.

Now a closer look at its many unique constituents:

$$CH_2=C_2H_3-\underset{O}{\overset{|}{S}}-\underset{NH_2}{\overset{|}{C}H_2}CH-COOH \quad \textbf{Allin}$$

$$C_3H_5-\underset{O}{\overset{|}{S}}-S-C_3H_5 \quad \textbf{Allicin}$$

2-propene-1-sulfinothioic acid S-2-propenyl ester

Allicin, garlic's natural antibiotic, is produced when garlic is chewed or ground. This action causes **allin** (or alliin, a sulfur-containing amino acid) to react with **allinase**, an enzyme contained in garlic. There are some evidence that the allicin concentration of fresh garlic extract actually increases over time as the enzymatic reaction continues to operate. This may account for the observations that aged extracts like Kyolic are more effective than fresh garlic for those properties affected by allicin.

Dr. Eugene Scnell is a chemist who has spent years researching herbal remedies in Japan and subsequently joined forces with Manji Wakunaga, a strong advocate of herbal medicine. Together, they perfected a 20-month aging process for cold-pressed whole garlic that allows the pungent and irritating allicin to undergo conversion to a nearly odorless form while enhancing many of its important pharmacological properties. In fact, the manufacturers of Kyolic brand aged garlic extract claim that their product contains up to seven times more of the herb's essential nutrients, including germanium and selenium.

Allicin has been demonstrated to block bacterial oxygen uptake by disrupting their cell membranes and interfering with lipid metabolism. Allicin also possesses anti-inflammatory properties and is the substance responsible for garlic's distinctive odor. Cooking garlic inactivates the heat-sensitive enzyme and prevents the formation of allicin. Consequently, cooked garlic is much milder in both smell and taste. Some advocates suggest that raw garlic should be used for its therapeutic rather than culinary benefits.

Closely related to allicin (by the removal of an oxygen molecule) is

$$C_3H_5-S-S-C_3H_5$$

Diallyl disulphide

Diallyl disulphide is the active metabolite of allicin which means that it is produced by the body once allicin is absorbed into the system. It comprises 60% of the essential garlic oil. This compound appears to be responsible for garlic's cholesterol- and lipid-lowering effects. The name of this compound emphasizes the fact that garlic contains one of the highest sulfur contents of all vegetables. It should not therefore be of any surprise that garlic excels as a natural antibiotic when organic sulfur is used as an effective antiseptic.

Isothiocyanic acid isobutyl ester (IAIE), dipropyl trisulfide (DPT), allyl mercapton (AM), Methyl propyl disulfide (MPD), propylene sulfide, dialkilsulfides, dithiins, adgoens, and **thioglycosidepeptides** are additional thiosulfinates with varying degrees of free-radical scavenging and antitumor effects.

Ajoene (4,5,9-trithiadodeca-1,6,11-triene-9-oxide is derived from the Spanish word for garlic, pronounced a-ho-een) was first identified by Dr. Eric Block, an organic chemist who has specialized in the study of garlic for 20 years at the State University of New York at Albany. Ajoene prevents red blood cells from sticking together and clumping into the dangerous blood clots that cause strokes and heart attacks.

This important compound is also involved in the body's ability to synthesize fat in such a way that it is able to very effectively control the production of cholesterol. This makes garlic especially useful in the prevention of atherosclerosis—hardening of the arteries. More recently ajoene has been found to be superior to allicin in its antifungal activity.

Yoshida, S., Kasunga, S., Hayashi, N., Ushiroguchi, T., Matsuura, H., Nakagawa, S. "Antifungal Activity of Ajoene Derived from Garlic" *Applied Environmental Microbiology* (53) 615, 1987.

Allithiamine is a biologically active form of vitamin B_1. It is formed by the coenzymatic action of vitamin B_1 on alliin as reported by Matzukawa in the *Journal of Pharmaceutical Society of Japan*, (72) 1585, 1952.

Selenium and **Germanium** are present in unusually high concentrations within the garlic clove and make garlic the best-known natural source of these trace elements. Garlic contains 9.3 grams of selenium per 100 grams of fresh bulb and 0.44 p.p.m. dry weight. Both selenium and germanium help protect cells from damaging oxidation and demonstrate a biological activity similar to vitamin E.

Oxidation, rusting of the body, is responsible for numerous disease processes including the aging process in general. Oxygen free radicals with unpaired electrons latch onto and damage other molecules, usually the lipid or fatty cell membranes. The rancidity of butter and nuts is a common example of fatty oxidation.

As a potent antioxidant, selenium counteracts the effects of harmful oxidizing substances that would otherwise break down cellular immunity and even contribute to cancer development. Loma Linda University researcher Dr. Benjamin Lau has reported that garlic "contains certain radical scavengers and may thus be useful for prevention of cancer."

Saponins are glycosides which appear to assist in lowering high blood pressure. They are named for the opalescent, frothy, soapy appearance they produce when mixed with water.

Fructans are carbohydrates that appear to stimulate the immune system and thus assist in preventing numerous diseases and pathological conditions.

Xyloglucans polysaccharide carbohydrates.

Bioflavonoids quercitin and cyanidin have also been identified.

Crotonaldehyde a bacteriocide and antiseptic.

Nutritional Contents per one pound

Calories	547	Iron	6.0 mg
Protein	24.8 g	Vitamin A	trace
Fat	.8 g	Thiamine	1.01 mg
Carbohydrates	123.0 g	Riboflavin	.31 mg
Calcium	116 mg	Niacin	1.9 mg
Phosphorus	806 mg	Vitamin C	59 mg

Antibiotic Properties

*"There appears to be sufficient data to indicate that
garlic is indeed a natural antibiotic...and holds a
promising position as a broad-spectrum therapeutic agent."*
Medical Hypotheses 12:227–37, 1983

Garlic has been popular for several thousand years as
an effective natural antibiotic and is still used today for the
treatment of infected wounds and skin ulcers by physicians
in India, China and Japan.

- The horrible Black Plague of the Middle Ages spared
  those who ate garlic daily.

- A garlic-vinegar preparation was credited with protecting many in the town of Marseilles, France during a 1722
  plague.

- Japanese researchers Amano and Kitagawa reported in
  1935 the antiseptic properties of garlic in treating the
  typhoid bacillus. In some cases it was shown to be more
  effective than penicillin.

Records from World War I include accounts of army
doctors who made use of garlic's ability to inhibit bacterial
growth. Field physicians soaked sterilized sphagnum moss
with garlic juice and applied the preparation to open
wounds. In 1916 the British government purchased many
tons of garlic at a shilling a pound for treating wounded
soldiers.

Starting in the 1970's a small flood of articles announcing the surprising antibiotic properties of garlic appeared in such diverse microbiology journals as

- *Planta Medica*
- *Review of Medical Virology*
- *Current Microbiology*
- *Mycopathology and Mycology Applications*
- *Mycologia*
- *Japanese Journal of Infectious Disease*
- *International Journal of Dermatology*

and more.

Equally impressive is the wide spectrum of garlic's antibiotic activity. *Allium* appears to be effective against such diverse pathological organisms as

- *Candida*
- *Histoplasma*
- *Cryptococcus*
- *Coccidiodes*
- *Sporotrichosis*
- *Tuberculosis*
- *Influenza B*
- *Herpes simplex*
- *AIDS virus*
- *Coxsackie,* and even
- *leprosy.*

A detailed review of specific literature references and anecdotal accounts follows.

Fungal Infections

Drs. Michael R. Tansey, J.A. Appleton, and F.E. Barone at Indiana University at Bloomington studied the effect of garlic on inhibiting the growth of mold and yeast.

Tansey, M.R.; Appleton, J.A., "Inhibition of Fungal Growth by Garlic Extract" Mycologia (67) 409, 1975.

Appleton, J.A.; Tansey, M.R., "Inhibition of Growth of Zoopathogenic Fungi by Garlic Extract" *Mycologia* (67) 882, 1975.

Barone, F.E., Tansey, M.R., "Isolation, Purification, Identification, Synthesis, and Kinetics of Activity of the Anticandidal Components of *Allium sativum* and a Hypothesis for its Mode of Action" *Mycologia* (69) 793, 1977.

Dr. Benjamin Lau and his graduate student, Moses Adetumbi, demonstrated the growth inhibiting ability of garlic against *Coccidioides immitis*, a mold responsible for causing Valley Fever in the western United States and a frequent opportunistic organism associated with AIDS victims.

Adetumbi, M.A., Lau, B.H.S., "Inhibition of In Vitro Germination and Spherulation of *Coccidioides immitis* by *Allium sativum*" Current Microbiology (13) 73, 1986.

Adetumbi determined that garlic exerted its antibiotic effects by interfering with lipid synthesis and thus impairing cell membrane operation. This, in turn, appeared to interfere with the yeast's ability to take up oxygen essentially leading to its asphyxiation.

Chicks infected with *Candida albicans* were successfully treated by feeding them garlic.

Prasad, G, Sharma, V.D, "Efficacy of Garlic (Allium sativum) Treatment Against Experimental Candidiasis in Chicks" *British Veterinary Journal* (136) 488, 1980.

Ringworm infested rabbits were treated with garlic, as well.

Amer, M., Taha, M., Tosson, Z. "The Effect of Aqueous Garlic Extract on the Growth of Dermatophytes" *International Journal of Dermatology* (19) 285, 1980.

Sporotrichosis is a particularly nasty fungal infection that invades the soft tissues and lymphatic channels after being inoculated in the affected human victim usually from rose thorn puncture wounds. Applying garlic extract to the ulcerations successfully cleared up the infection.

Tutakne, M.A., Bhardwaj, J.R., Satyanarayanan, G, Sethi, I.C. "Sporotrichosis Treated with Garlic Juice" *Indian Journal of Dermatology* (28) 40, 1983.

Viral Infections

Garlic has been shown to exhibit antiviral activity against influenza, herpes simplex, and coxsackie viruses by inhibiting the virus's multiplication.

Tsai, Y., Cole, L.L., Davis, L.E., Lockwood, S.J., Simmons, V., and Wild, G.C. "Antiviral Properties of Garlic: In Vitro Effects on Influenza B, Herpes simplex and Coxsackie Viruses" *Planta Medica* (5) 460, 1985.

Garlic was shown to reduce the severity of influenza virus infections in mice.

Esanu, V. Prahoveanu, E. "The Effect of Garlic Extract, Applied as such or in Association with NaF, on Experimental Influenza in Mice" *Reviews in Romanian Medical Virology* (34) 11, 1983.

And garlic appears to also beef up the production of antibodies in animals who are immunized with influenza vaccines.

Nagai, K. "Experimental Studies on the Preventive Effect of Garlic Extract Against Infection with Influenza Virus" *Japanese Journal of Infectious Disease* (47) 321, 1973.

Human cytomegalovirus (HCMV) is stopped dead in its tracks when it tries to tangle with garlic. N.L. Guo, et al, demonstrated garlic's amazing anti-viral talents in a 1993 issue of the Clinical Medicine Journal. They used tissue cultures to measure the size of viral colonies developing with and without the presence of garlic extract. The virus was inhibited in direct proportion to the garlic dose. But the greatest protection was achieved if they *pretreated* the tissue culture with garlic *before* virus exposure and then maintained a continuous effective concentration thereafter.

Guo, N.L., Lu, D.P., Woods, G.L., Reed, E., Zhou, G.Z., Zhang, L.B., Waldman, R.H. "Demonstration of the anti-viral activity of garlic extract against human cytomegalovirus in vitro" *Chin Med J* (Engl) (1993 Feb) 106(2):93–6

Oral Disease

Allicin has been shown to posses an antibiotic effectiveness that is equivalent to penicillin. Remember, of course, that penicillin was first discovered in a number of different fruit molds. But garlic appears to have a much wider application and is not limited by any known allergenic risks. Ironically, however, it has been shown to be effective in treating the nasty bad breath of halitosis by eliminating the offending oral bacteria from gingivitis and tooth decay. A mouthwash prepared from a 10 percent garlic extract results in a dramatic reduction in the problematic oral flora.

Respiratory Conditions

Dr. Carl Fliermans at the University of Kentucky in Lexington showed how garlic was a potent inhibitor of the pulmonary fungal pathogen *Histoplasma capsulatum*.

Fliermans, C.B.: "Inhibition of *Histoplasma capsulatum* by garlic." *Mycopathology and Mycological Applications* (50)227, 1973.

Dr. Edward Delaha and Vincent Garagusi of George Washington University in Washington D.C. reported that garlic inhibited the growth of many acid-fast bacteria including species that cause both tuberculosis and leprosy.

Delaha, E.C., Garagusi, V.F. "Inhibition of Mycobacteria by Garlic Extract (*Allium sativum*)" *Antimicrobial Agents and Chemotherapy* (27) 485, 1985.

Tuberculosis has been treated by inhaling steam containing garlic oil or garlic juice. In the former Soviet Union garlic is called 'Russian penicillin.' During a recent influenza outbreak, officials used 500 tons of garlic in managing the wide-scale epidemic.

Garlic has been shown to act as an expectorant, causing mucus production to change to a more easily eliminated thin, watery serous secretion. Russian researchers use a mixture of garlic and sunflower oil as an aromatic chest rub in treating pediatric sinusitis and pertussis or whooping cough cases.

Garlic also possesses a bronchodilating effect that is beneficial in treating asthma and bronchitis. More simple problems such as a sore-throat or nasal congestion respond to swallowing a teaspoon of garlic syrup made from squeezing the juice from a few cloves into honey.

Swimmer's Ear is an infection of the ear canal usually triggered by trapped water, not only from swimming, but bathing as well. These infections are usually bacterial, but a few are caused by fungal organisms. Commercially available agents are available, but significant side effects (like ototoxicity leading to hearing loss) limit their long term use. And if the ear drum is perforated these preparations may be actually contraindicated. A 1995 study comparing the antifungal properties of various pharmaceutical preparations and commercial garlic supplements looked at the genus Aspergillus, probably the most common cause of chronic otomycosis. They found that aqueous garlic extract and concentrated garlic oil were equal to or better than the prescription drugs.

> Pai, S.T., Platt, M.W. "Antifungal effects of Allium sativum (garlic) extract against the Aspergillus species involved in otomycosis" *Lett Appl Microbiol* (1995 Jan) 20(1):14–8

Frequent mention of garlic's use as a topical antibiotic for external otitis is encountered worldwide. Oral garlic works just as effectively for this disorder.

A Case History

An elderly lady whom I met living in upstate New York near the Canadian border recounted for me her experience with garlic. She suddenly began to develop recurring external otitis affecting her right ear while in her sixth decade of life. She suffered 13 flare-ups in a single year. She didn't experience any discharge or fever; just pain and some swelling of her ear canal. Her physician prescribed various neosporin-polymixin- or gentamycin-based antibiotic ear drops. She would experience temporary relief but her symptoms of pain and swelling promptly returned as soon as these preparations were discontinued. This stubbornly chronic ailment began to suggest the possibility of a fungal infection and prescription medication for this was tried as well but without success. Then a friend suggested garlic. She began to take 1,500 mg garlic oil capsules twice a day and experienced a prompt resolution of her problem. She has not had any further recurrence for the following ten years. And, as a side benefit, she has noticed that she has not had any of her usually annual 'colds' or bouts of flu.

As early as 1897, the absorption of garlic through the skin was known to produce its characteristic odor during exhalation. An account of this phenomenon was recorded by W.T. Fernie, M.D. in his book *Herbal Simples.*

> "The odour of the bulb is very diffusible, even when it is aplied to the soles of the feet its odour is exhaled by the lungs."

This observation was not isolated. Repeated accounts of using garlic cloves placed inside walking shoes appear in the literature. The aromatic oils are released as the cloves are crushed and are quickly absorbed through the skin into the circulation.

> "If chopped or minced fresh garlic is placed on the soles of the feet and allowed to remain there for some time, it will not be long before the odor of garlic can be detected on the breath; and cases of purulent disease in different parts of the body have been reported completely cured by simply keeping an application of garlic to the soles of the feet, and renewing it once or twice a day."
>
> *Advanced Treatise in Herbology*, E.E. Shook

This is a novel route of administration reminiscent of DSMO's heyday as a potential topical drug vehicle.

Meningitis

Dr. Robert A. Fromtling when at the University of Oklahoma, demonstrated the growth inhibiting effect of garlic on *Cryptococcus neoformans*, a yeast which can cause a serious and frequently fata form of meningitis.

Fromtling, R., Bulmer, G.S. "In vitro Effect of Aqueous Extract of Garlic (*Allium sativum*) on the Growth and Viability of *Cryptococcus neoformans*" *Mycologia* (70) 397, 1978.

Fromtling's observations were confirmed by a 1994 report which pitted the relative effectiveness of garlic against amphotericin B, the mainline intravenous antifungal drug used in the treatment of cryptococcal meningitis. The researchers, lead by L.E. Davis, found that concentrated garlic extract has potent fungistatic and fungicidal activity. They could stifle the growth of 100,000 cryptococci with only 6 micrograms of garlic extract in a single cubic centimeter of water. But more than that, they found that when they used both garlic and amphotericin B, the antifungal effect was much more than simply the additive effects of each agent. Garlic appears to potentiate and enhance the activity of amphotericin B.

Davis, L.E., Shen, J., Royer, R.E. "In vitro synergism of concentrated *Allium sativum* extract and amphotericin B against *Cryptococcus neoformans*" *Planta Med* (1994 Dec) 60(6):546–9

A University of New Mexico School of Medicine study delivered garlic extract by intravenous injection directly into the blood stream to five patients with **meningitis**, two of which had a **cryptococcal** fungal form of the infection. Four out of the five patients demonstrated a significant drop in the concentration of fungal spores in their CSF (cerebrospinal fluid) after treatment. It was credited with an 82% cure rate for fungal meningitis as compared with only 15% for Amphetericin B. *BEPHA Bulletin*, July 1986.

Hunan Medical College in the People's Republic of China successfully treated eleven of 21 cases of Cryptococcal meningitis with oral, intramuscular and intravenous injections of garlic over a period of several weeks.

> Hunan Medical College, China "Garlic in Cryptococcal Meningitis. A Preliminary Report of 21 Cases" *Chinese Medical Journal* (93) 123, 1980.

Physicians in Singapore reported similar experience with both garlic and conventional medications.

> Tjia, T.L., Yeow, Y.K., Tan, C.B. "Cryptococcal Meningitis" *Journal of Neurology and Neurosurgical Psychology* (48) 853, 1985.

Polio

Several articles in the *Antibiotics Annal* over the years 1958 and 1959 reported a 30% reduction in incidence for poliomyelitis in patients who were treated with garlic over an untreated control group.

Herpes

Utah's Brigham Young University conducted research that showed the complete inactivation of herpes simplex virus types 1 and 2 by the use of fresh garlic extract.

Parasites

The Swiss Tropical Institute found that "the [garlic] compound has the potential to be used for treatment of several human and animal parasitic diseases."

Ajoene, best known for its anti-clotting effects, is also an effective antibiotic against *Trypanosoma cruzi*, the protazoal organism which causes **Chagas' disease**. The way it operates in this situation was reported by the journal of Biochemical Pharmacology in 1993. Ajoene was shown to interfere with lipid production, and lipids are critical for the fabrication of cell membrane structures. Extremely low concentrations of Ajoene will immediately arrest the development of Trypanosomal intermediate stages and higher concentrations weaken the cell walls to the point that the parasites literally explode.

> Urbina, J.A., Marchan, E., Lazardi, K., Visbal, G., Apitz-Castro, R., Gil, F., Aguirre, T., Piras, M.M., Piras, R. "Inhibition of phosphatidylcholine biosynthesis and cell proliferation in Trypanosoma cruzi by ajoene, an antiplatelet compound isolated from garlic" *Biochem Pharmacol* (1993 Jun 22) 45(12):2381–7

A medical student from Tufts University, while conducting research during a summer session at Israel's Weizmann Institute, heard an interesting story from a Peace Corps volunteer regarding the use of garlic in treating local maladies. Further investigation showed that garlic stopped the growth of Entamoeba histolytica, the parasite responsible for millions of cases of dysentery worldwide every year.

> Varon, S. "Medical Student Discovers Curative Powers of Garlic" *Heritage*, April 10, 1987, p. 28.

Insecticide

In addition to garlic's amazing antibiotic effects, numerous accounts of its use in controlling fleas, ticks and mosquitoes exist. For example, volatile fractions of both aqueous and alcoholic extracts of garlic have been used to treat pets and livestock infested with ticks, killing them within 30 minutes and repelling new infestations. G. Catar, *Bratislav. lekarske Listy*, (34) 1004, 1954.

Staph

A 1994 article in the *Journal of Applied Bacteriology* reported the effectiveness of garlic in squelching the growth of Staphylococcus aureus and its nasty enterotoxins.

Gonzalez-Fandos, E., Garcia-Lopez, M.L., Sierra, M.L., Otero, A. "Staphylococcal growth and enterotoxins (A-D) and thermonuclease synthesis in the presence of dehydrated garlic" *J Appl Bacteriol* (1994 Nov) 77(5):549–52

Gastrointestinal Disorders

Old Dr. Fernie in another of his books, *Meals Medicinal*, advised that "a garlic clove, when introduced into the bowel, will destroy thread worms, and, if eaten, will abolish round worms." But this was old news indeed, because garlic has been extolled for this purpose since ancient times by Babylonians, Hindus, Chinese, Greeks and Romans.

A published article by F. Damrau and E.A. Ferguson in *Reviews of Gastroenterology* (16) 411, 1949 identified another compound called *allichalon* which has a sedating action on gastric motility.

While consuming more garlic has definite health benefits, you don't want to overdo it. As an antibiotic, garlic can tear up the gastrointestinal system. Raw garlic can be toxic if taken in unreasonably large quantities and has been reported to cause gastrointestinal irritation. Cooked garlic or processed extracts such as the Kyolic brand, will avoid this.

Nakagawa, S., et al "Effect of raw and extracted-aged garlic juice on growth of young rats and their organs after peroral administration" *Journal of Toxicological Science* (5) 91, 1980.

Hemorrhoids

Garlic suppositories (peeled cloves, sliced down the sides) will produce curative results when steroids and other highly touted remedies fail. I have personally witnessed this overnight miracles in a patient with stubborn bleeding internal lesions after a single application.

Cardiovascular Benefits

French scientists first noticed the cardiovascular benefits of Mediterranean diets. People living in this part of the world enjoy a low incidence of heart disease because they use very little saturated fat from their abundant supply of olives and a large amount of fresh vegetables including garlics.

Good Cholesterol

Cholesterol has gotten a considerable amount of bad press in recent years, but it does have an important place within the human body. Cholesterol forms the basis of cell membranes, vital hormones, and electrical insulation around most of the body's nerve fibers. Our system normally produces around 2,000 mg every day to meet these needs. But too much of a good thing spells trouble. And that's exactly what the average American adult faces when he or she daily consumes nearly 500 mg of additional cholesterol.

Cholesterol travels through our blood streams in two basic forms. High density lipoproteins (HDL) scrub down excess cholesterol from the walls of our arteries and transport it to the liver where it can be removed from the body. HDL is 'good cholesterol' and higher levels (than the other form) are *highly* desirable.

But the other form, low density lipoprotein (LDL) are tiny packages of cholesterol that can easily slip through an artery's thin lining to collect and buildup into what may one day block the flow of blood. Reducing the relative amount of LDL and the total amount of *both* types of cholesterol is important in preventing heart attacks and strokes.

Two published reports by Asaf A. Qureshi, research chemist at the U.S. Department of Agriculture's Barley and Malt Laboratory discovered that odorless water-soluble components of garlic were as equally effective in lowering lipids as smelly allicin.

Qureshi, A.A., Din, Z.Z., Abuirmeileh, N., Burger, W.C., Ahman, Y., Elson, C.E. "Suppression of Avian Hepatic Lipid Metabolism by Solvent Extracts of Garlic: Impact on serum lipids" *Journal of Nutrition* (113) 1746, 1983.
Qureshi, A.A., et al "Inhibition of Cholesterol and Fatty Acid Biosynthesis in Liver Enzymes and Chicken Hepatocytes by Polar Fractions of Garlic" *Lipids* (18) 343, 1983.

The Clinical Research Center in New Orleans examined the cholesterol levels of 42 healthy middle-aged men and women and found an average of 262 mg per 100 ml of blood or 262 mg%. The group was divided and half received a 300mg garlic powder tablet three times a day. The other half received an identically appearing placebo tablet three times a day as well. After 12 weeks the garlic group dropped their cholesterol levels down to 247mg%. There was no statistically significant change in the placebo group.

The Department of Medicine at the New York Medical College reported in the journal *Annals of Internal Medicine* that merely "one-half to one clove [of garlic] a day or its equivalent may decrease total serum cholesterol levels by about 9 percent," a figure which they considered "conservative."

An Oxford University study in England reviewed the results of 16 previous studies involving 952 patients. Cholesterol levels were reduced by those taking garlic preparations by an average of 12 percent—and remained at the reduced level six months later. They concluded that "garlic supplements may have an important role to play in the treatment of hypercholesterolaemia" (high cholesterol blood levels).

German experiments showed even greater promise. In seven out of eight studies involving over 500 subjects, daily garlic powder supplementation dropped the cholesterol levels from 5 to 20 percent. They found that eating garlic appeared to actually prevent fat digestion, allowing a reduction of cholesterol even when subjects did *not* adhere to a strict low-fat diet.

French researches have identified that one of garlic's key ingredients, ajoene, appears to inhibit the production of human gastric lipase (HGL), an enzyme which the body produces to digest and absorb dietary fat. "These data may explain the age-old Mediterranean and Oriental belief in the 'blood-thinning' effects of garlic on a molecular and physiologic basis," they concluded.

Garlic not only lowers the overall cholesterol level, but makes a shift in the HDL:LDL ratio that is also beneficial. It lowers the vessel-clogging LDL while raising the vessel-cleaning HDL levels.

Furthermore, new evidence strongly suggests that garlic not only decreases cholesterol production, but assists in shifting cholesterol from tissue stores into the blood stream for an even more important reduction of total *body* cholesterol. Simply looking at serum cholesterol levels may not always tell the whole story. Although chronic static serum levels may associate well with atherosclerotic risk, interpretation of changing levels depends on the direction of tissue:serum shifts.

This was first observed by Dr. Arun Bordia while studying the effects of garlic supplementation on lipid levels in patients with coronary heart disease. He recorded an initial paradoxical rise in blood lipid levels after starting garlic therapy. See figure 1.

> Bordia, A. "Effect of Garlic on Blood Lipids in Patients with Coronary Heart Disease" *American Journal of Clinical Nutrition* (34) 2100, 1981.

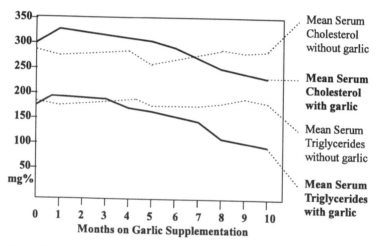

Long Term Comparison of Serum Lipids on the Effect of Garlic
—Figure 1—

Benjamin Lau and two of his clinical colleagues conducted a similar study on blood lipid response to odorless Kyolic garlic extract. They divided their experiment into three parts. Part One involved two groups of 16 subjects with a history of elevated cholesterol levels. The first group received four Kyolic garlic extract capsules daily. The other group received an identically appearing placebo. The results of both cholesterol and triglyceride concentrations in their test subjects is shown in figure 2.

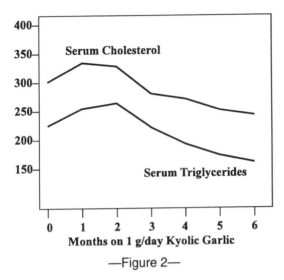

—Figure 2—

Lau and his group also observed an initial rise of both cholesterol and triglyceride levels in those patients who received garlic. Although they were disappointed at first, as they continued the experiment levels in the garlic group ultimately dropped well below the control group. This confirmed the experience of Dr. Bordia and his theory that such data was demonstrating the migration of sequestered lipids *out* of tissue deposits *into* the blood stream.

Part Two studied a group of fourteen subjects with normal serum lipid levels. The results were as expected: both placebo and garlic groups had similar lipids levels at the end of the study. But once again, those taking garlic experienced an initial rise in their cholesterol and triglyceride levels during the first two months.

The final Part Three of the Lau study again involved patients with elevated cholesterols. This time, however, they looked at high- and low-density lipoprotein levels. Those taking garlic experienced an initial rise in both LDL and VLDL levels that closely paralleled the total cholesterol levels observed in Part One of the study. Later in the ne levels of HDL in the garlic supplemented group gan to increase, though much less dramatically than the sudden surge of the LDLs. Garlic appeared to be "flushing out" the "bad" cholesterol and then stimulating the production of "good" cholesterol.

The Bordia theory has been validated by a number of independent studies. Researchers at the U.S. Department of Agriculture's Nutrition Institute found fewer lipid deposits in the liver of rats who had been fed garlic extract for eighteen days. But measurements of their blood serum lipids were significantly higher. See figure 3.

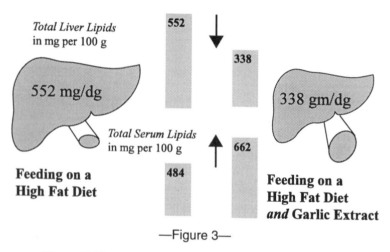

—Figure 3—

Chang, M.L, Johnson, M.A. "Effect of Garlic on Carbohydrate Metabolism and Lipid Synthesis in Rats" *Journal of Nutrition* (110) 931, 1980.

See also:

Chi, M.S., Koh, E.T., Stewart, T.J. "Effects of Garlic on Lipid Metabolism in Rats Fed Cholesterol or Lard" *Journal of Nutrition* (112) 241, 1982.
Jain, R.C. "Onion and Garlic in Experimental Cholesterol Atherosclerosis in Rabbits. I. Effect of serum lipids and development of atherosclerosis" *Artery* (1) 115, 1975.

Nakamura, H., Ishikawa, M. "Effect of
S-methyl-1-cysteine sulfoxide on Cholesterol Metabolism"
Kanzo (12) 673, 1971.
Kritchevsky, D., Tepper, S.A., Morisey, R., Klurfeld, D.
"Influence of Garlic Oil on Cholesterol Metabolism in
Rats" *Nutrition Reports International* (22) 641, 1980.

On August 28–30, 1991 the U.S. Department of Agriculture and Pennsylvania State University cosponsored the First Annual Congress on the Health Significance of Garlic and Garlic Constituents in Washington, D.C. Among the many reports was that of Dr. David Kritchevsky from the Wistar Institute in Philadelphia. His study of laboratory rabbits with induced atherosclerosis showed a reduction in blood vessel blockage (vascular occlusion) by as much as 31 percent when these animals were fed a diet containing corn and garlic oils.

High Blood Pressure

Reports of the beneficial uses of garlic in controlling hypertension were published as early as 1921.

Loeper, M. Debray, M. "Antihypertensive Action of Garlic
Extract" *Bulletin of the Society of Medicine* (37) 1032,
1921.

Dr. F. G. Piotrowski at the University of Geneva, Switzerland, observed a vasodilating effect [dilation of the blood vessels] while using garlic to reduce blood pressure in 100 of his hypertensive patients. He observed a drop of 20 mmHg in blood pressure in 40% of these cases after a week of garlic treatment.

Piotrowski, F.G. "L'ail en therapeutique" *Praxis*, July 1,
1948, p. 488.

Bulgarian researcher V. Petkov published numerous articles on his experiments involving animals and humans on the effects of garlic in reducing high blood pressure. For example:

"A Pharmacological Study of Garlic (Allium sativum L.)" *Annuaire de l'Universite de Sofia, Faculte de Medecine*, t. XXVIII 885, 1949.
"On the Action of Garlic (Allium sativum L.) on the Blood Pressure" *Sovremenna Medizina* (1) 5, 1950.
"New Experimental Data about the Pharmocodynamics of Some Plant Species" *Sofia: Nauka I Iskustve* 227, 1953.
"Uber die Pharmakodynamik einiger in Bulgarien wildwashsender bzw angebauter Arzneipflanzen" *Zeitschreift fur arztliche Fortbildung* (56) 430, 1962.

V. Petkov studied the effects of garlic on reducing blood pressure on 114 patients with hypertension and atherosclerosis. His findings were reported in the German pharmaceutical journal Deutche Apotheker-Z., 106(51), p. 1861, 1966. Garlic produced a reduction in systolic pressure from 8–33 mmHg and diastolic from 4–20 mmHg.

Petkov injected fresh garlic juice intravenously into cats and recorded only slight and, even then, only temporary decreases in blood pressure. But when when the prepared garlic juice had been stored for seven to twelve months, he observed a significantly increased effect. He concluded that aged garlic extract provided time for an enzymatic process or processes to release active components not available in fresh preparations.

Two studies on a smaller scale were reported in the Britich Medical Journal, Lancet, in 1969.

Papayannopoulos, G. "Garlic" Lancet (2) 962, 1969.
Srinivasan, V. "A new Antihypertensive Agent" *Lancet* (2) 800, 1969.

The experience of Drs. Sainani, Desai, and More was reported in the Canadian Journal of Health and Nutrition,

Number 12, 1977. They demonstrated the beneficial results of garlic and onions have on both high blood pressure and heart disease.

Drs. Sainani and Desai also published several additional articles on the cardiovascular benefits of garlic and onion as observed in the Indian community of Jain. They reported that those who ate garlic as a regular part of their diet demonstrated not only **lower cholesterol and triglycerides**, but **lower fibrinogen, a longer clotting time**, and an **ability to break up clots** that was superior to those who did not eat garlic.

Sainani, G.S., Desai, D.B., Gorhe, N.H., Natu, S.M., Pise, D.V., Sainani, P.G. "Dietary Garlic, Onion and Some Coagulation Parameters in Jain Community" *Journal of the Association of Physicians in India* (27) 707, 1979.
Sainani, G.S., Desai, D.B., Gorhe, N.H., Natu, S.M., Pise, D.V., Sainani, P.G. "Effect of Dietary Garlic and Onion on Serum Lipid Profile in Jain Community" *Indian Journal of Medical Research* (69) 776, 1979.
Sainani, G.S., Desai, D.B., More, K.N. "Onion, Garlic and Atherosclerosis" *Lancet* (1) 575, 1976.

Patients with severely elevated blood pressures were studied at the Clinical Research Center in New Orleans. Nine patients receiving 2,400 mg of garlic demonstrated a nearly immediate drop in their pressure. Within five hours after this single dose, some pressures had fallen by nearly 50 percent.

Dr. Bolton, Professor of Pharmacy at St. John's University College of Pharmacy and Allied Health Professions in Jamaica, New York published an historical summary of the uses of garlic. He noted that garlic has been used for treating hypertension in China and Japan for centuries. Garlic is officially recognized for this use by the Japanese Food and Drug Administration.

Bolton, S., Null, G., Troetel, W.M. "The Medical Uses of Garlic—Fact and Fiction" *American Pharmacology* (22) 448, 1985.

A 1973 study in China involved 70 hypertensive patients who were treated with 50 grams of raw garlic a day. They observed an overall positive response in nearly 62%. Nearly half in the study, 33 patients, showed a marked lowering of the blood pressure; and 14 showed moderate reductions.

Bordia, A., Bansal, H.C. "Essential Oil of Garlic in Prevention of Atherosclerosis" Lancet (2) 1491, 1973. Zheziang Institute of Traditional Chinese Medicine: "The effect of essential oil of garlic on hyperlipemia and platelet aggregation" *Journal of Traditional Chinese Medicine* (6) 117, 1986.

A 1994 study by Y. Ozturk and friends demonstrated that garlic exercises its blood pressure lowering effect by relaxing the muscle layer of blood vessels.

Ozturk, Y., Aydin, S., Kosar, M., Baser, K.H. "Endothelium-dependent and independent effects of garlic on rat aorta." *J Ethnopharmacol* (1994 Oct) 44(2):109–16

Anti-Clotting

Recent advances in pharmacological research have produced a number of platelet inhibitors. This class of drugs is important in reducing the risk of clot formation. Aspirin, the first and most commonly used drug for this purpose, is still widely used. But aspirin and even the newer compounds have significant side effects that limit and sometimes prevent their use in some patients. Garlic contains ajoene, the substance responsible for its strong odor. Dr. Eric Block, who first isolated ajoene, considers it to be as effective as aspirin in the prevention of blood clots.

Block, E., Ahmad, S., Mahendra, J.K., Crecely, R.W., Apitz-Castro, R., Cruz, M.R. "Ajoene: a Potent Antithrombotic Agent from Garlic" *Journal of the American Chemical Society* (106) 8295, 1984.

An Italian study showed that taking 900 mg of garlic powder daily produced a significant reduction in blood clotting function within seven to 14 days.

Garlic was used in a study on patients with **claudication**. They had narrowing and near obstruction of the blood vessels in their legs which caused disabling pain when they walked over 100 meters. After they had taken 800mg a day of garlic powder tablets for 12 weeks they averaged a 15 meter increase in their walking distance. Even after 5 weeks of treatment there was a noticeable drop in their diastolic blood pressure and plasma viscosity (thickness). In addition they displayed a significantly lower rate of spontaneous thrombocyte aggregation (less tendency to form clots).

Kiesewetter, H., Jung, F., Jung, E.M., Blume, J., Mrowietz, C., Birk, A., Koscielny, J., Wenzel, E. "Effects of garlic coated tablets in peripheral arterial occlusive disease" *Clin Investig* (1993 May) 71(5):383–6

Aged garlic extract was used in a study presented at the 1993 meeting of the American Association of Cancer Research. Bovine pulmonary arteries (arteries from the lungs of cows) were exposed to hydrogen peroxide and the **oxidative damage on the endothelium** (cells which form the inside lining of the blood vessel) was measured. Cells which had been preincubated with the garlic extract overnight could withstand any damage from the hydrogen peroxide even after a three hour exposure.

Yamasaki, T., Li, L., Lau, B.H. "Garlic extract protects vascular endothelial cells from oxidant injury" (Meeting abstract) *Proc Annu Meet Am Assoc Cancer Res* (1993) 34:A3299 1993

Antioxidant

Vitamins C, E and A gained a certain amount of notoriety as antioxidants, important in the prevention of oxygen free-radical formation. In respect to garlic's antioxidant qualities, the aqueous extract obtained from **1mg of the garlic preparation** has been found to have the **anti-oxidative effectiveness of 30 nmol of ascorbic acid (vitamin C)** and/or **3.6 nmol of alpha-tocopherol (vitamin E)**.

Popov, I., Blumstein, A., Lewin, G. "Antioxidant effects of aqueous garlic extract. 1st communication: Direct detection using the photochemiluminescence" *Arzneimittelforschung* (1994 May) 44(5):602–4

Antiarrythmic

Garlic is also able to calm an irritable heart. German investigators Isensee, Rietz and Jacob showed that garlic protected mammalian hearts against the development of dangerous rhythms. They tied off a branch of the main coronary artery in rat hearts and then watched for ventricular tachycardia or fibrillation. This was the physiological equivalent of producing an experimental heart attack. With blood flow interrupted, oxygen levels in the heart muscle supplied by the coronary artery dropped quickly. Under normal conditions 35% of the hearts would go into ventricular tachycardia within 20 minutes; 88% would develop fatal fibrillation.

When they changed the rat's diets to include 1% garlic powder, their susceptibility to these rhythms (after 10 weeks of treatment) dropped dramatically. None of the garlic-fed hearts developed ventricular tachycardia and fibrillation dropped to a 50% incidence. Even then, it took longer to develop and the duration was shortened. See figure 4.

Isensee, H., Rietz, B., Jacob, R. "Cardioprotective actions of garlic (Allium sativum)" *Arzneimittelforschung* (1993 Feb) 43(2):94–8

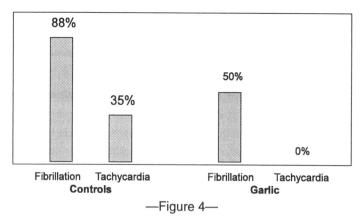

—Figure 4—

Immunotherapy and Cancer

Garlic has consistently demonstrated impressive anti-mutagenic and anti-neoplastic effects. See the *American Journal of Chinese Medicine* 11:69–73, *Science* 126:1112–14, *Journal of Urology* 136:701–705; 137:359–62. This would seem to support some anecdotal accounts of its success in treating conditions like psoriasis where there is excessively rapid cell turnover.

In 1957 researcher A.S. Weisberger reported the tumor inhibiting capabilities of garlic and attributed this to the inactivation of certain sulfhydryl compounds present in tumor cells.

Weisberger, A.S., Pensky, J. "Tumor-inhibiting effects derived from an active principle of garlic (*Allium sativum*)" *Science* (126) 1112, 1957.

Weisberger, A.S., Pensky, J. "Tumor inhibition by a sulfhydril-blocking agent related to an active princple of garlic (*Allium sativum*)" *Cancer Research* (18) 1301, 1958.

Dr. Lau has also participated in the beneficial effects of odorless garlic extract in the treatment of bladder cancer. His conclusion: "Allium sativum was shown to elicit macrophages and lymphocytes [cells which attack cancer] leading to cytotoxic destruction of tumor cells." The tests were conducted with the assistance of several urologists who looked at the effect of locally injecting live BCG vaccine, killed *Corynebacterium parvum* vaccine, and liquid garlic extract on their bladder cancer patients. Garlic and the killed vaccine produced much greater tumor size reduction than the live BCG vaccine. In fact, after five alternate day treatments, the garlic and killed vaccine subjects showed no tumor cells on microscopic examination—only scar tissue. See figure 5.

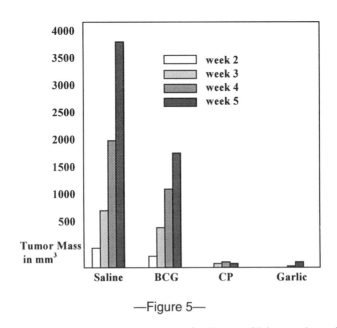

—Figure 5—

Dr. Keith Block, director of a large Chicago hospital oncology unit believes garlic "is an incredibly powerful agent and has immense physiological and clinical benefits." He recommends six to ten cloves of garlic daily as an immunity-booster.

John Wayne Cancer Institute in Santa Monica, California found that garlic extract improved the cancer-fighting capacity of lymphocytes against leukemia.

Tests by Dr. Tariq Abdullah, a Florida pathologist, were designed to measure the effectiveness of macrophage killer cells in attacking cultured tumor cells. The study involved three groups of volunteers. The first group took 500mg of raw garlic every day per kg of body weight. The second group took 1.8 g of Kyolic garlic extract daily. And the third group used no garlic preparations and served as controls. At the end of three weeks, blood samples from each volunteer were prepared and exposed to the tumor cell cultures. The natural killer cells from the first group who ate raw garlic were able to destroy nearly 140% more tumor cells than the control group who ate no garlic. But the group treated with Kyolic garlic showed nearly 160% better tumor cell killing ability.

> Kandil, O.M., Abdullah, T.H., Elkadi, A. "Garlic and the immune system in humans: its effect on natural killer cells" *Federation Proceedings* (46) 441, 1987.

N. Monoka and team reported on another component of garlic in the October 1993 issue of *Cancer Immunology and Immunotherapy*. They studied the effect of a protein fraction which they isolated from aged garlic extract called Fraction 4 or simply F4. This garlic protein significantly enhanced the ability of human lymphocytes to seek and destroy tumor cells. And it appeared to synergize the potency of interleukin-2, even in suboptimal doses.

> Morioka, N., Sze, L.L. Morton, D.L., Irie, R.F. "A protein fraction from aged garlic extract enhances cytotoxicity and proliferation of human lymphocytes mediated by interleukin-2 and concanavalin A" *Cancer Immunol Immunother* (1993 Oct) 37(5):316–22

AIDS

The immunotherapeutic use of garlic in the treatment of cancer raises the possibility of additional applications. Human Immunodeficiency Virus infections are associated with the development of certain cancers, leukemias and lymphomas. The propspect was considered that garlic might also improve the immune status of patients infected with the AIDS virus.

Researchers at the Akbar Research Foundation in Panama City, Florida found that garlic could significantly improve the immune response of seven out of 10 AIDS patients. They administered five grams daily of an aged garlic extract (SGP) for six weeks, followed by 10 grams daily for an additional six week period.

Free Radical Scavenger

Studies at Beijing College in China and Greece have confirmed the LLUMC research that garlic contains potent free radical scavengers and is very effective in preventing the carcinogenic effects of *in vitro* oxidation. A study at the University of Kansas Medical Center involved ten healthy volunteers who received 600 mg of garlic powder daily for two weeks. They observed a 34 percent reduction in oxidation damage on their red blood cells after treatment.

The high levels of **selenium** in garlic is responsible for the herb's remarkable antioxidant properties. Selenium is a constituent of *glutathione peroxidase* (GSH-Px), an enzyme which prevents the formation of free radicals. The antitumor properties observed in selenium may result from its ability to chemically replace the sulfur molecule in L-cystine. This amino acid is consumed at high rates inside leukemic white blood cells. Selenium-modified L-cystine is able to suppress the growth of leukemia in animal studies.

University of Miami School of Medicine research has shown a correlation between low blood levels of GSH-Px and cancer patients living in selenium-poor parts of the world. In contrast to these findings, they also discovered that exceptionally low rates of stomach, liver, and esophageal cancer are observed in areas where soil concentrations of selenium are high. As a result of this, China has engaged in the practice of actually spraying selenium on farm crops as a public health program to prevent cancer in certain high-risk areas.

The American Health Foundation in Valhalla, New York reports that raising garlic in selenium-fertilized soil increases its natural selenium content and enhances its natural anti-carcinogenic abilities. The foundation has concluded that "the incorporation of selenium into garlic, which contains an abundant source of a variety of cancer-fighting sulfur compounds, may enhance its potential attributes in cancer protection."

The Roswell Park Cancer Institute in Buffalo, New York has also reported that "garlic expressed good anti-cancer activity" and has proposed that the general public could be immunized against cancer through the use of garlic-mediated "chemoprevention." They also advised the mass cultivation of 'designer foods' like garlic grown in selenium-enriched soil.

Their research investigated the protective effects of garlic against the development of **breast cancer** in laboratory mice. While regular garlic powder showed significantly less tumor formation, selenium-rich garlic produced the fewest number of mammary tumors.

The same story was told in a paper presented at the 1993 Annual Meeting of the Association of Cancer Researchers. Reporting on yet another example of the selenium-garlic-sulfur-cancer connection, the authors expressed their conviction that the organoselenium compounds in garlic are superior to their organosulfur equivalents in the prevention of tumors and cancer. They found that **diallyl selenide** (DASe) was about 300 times more anticarcinogenic than diallyl sulfide (DAS) in inhibiting the development of chemically induced **breast tumors** in rats.

El-Bayoumy, K., Ip, C., Chae, Y.H., Upadhyaya, P., Lisk, D., Prokopczyk, B. "Mammary cancer chemoprevention by diallyl selenide, a novel organoselenium compound" (Meeting abstract) *Proc Annu Meet Am Assoc Cancer Res* (1993) 34:A3322 1993

Nitrate Scavenger

Garlic also has gained recognition for containing **sulphydryl compounds** like allicin. Sulphydryl compounds are of great value in blocking the formation of **nitrosamines**, potent carcinogenic compounds used as preservatives in meats like sausages and ham.

An interesting epidemiological study conducted in China compared two large populations in the Shandong Province. Residents of Cangshan County enjoyed an exceptionally low death rate from **stomach cancer**: only 3 per 100,000 deaths. A second county, Oixia, has a thirteenfold higher death rate of 40 per 100,000. Researchers interviewed 1131 controls and 564 patients with gastric carcinomas and learned that Cangshan residents consumed 20 grams of garlic per day on average while those living in Oixia rarely eat garlic. Further study by gastric analysis showed very low concentrations of nitrites in those from Cangshan.

Mei, X., Wang, M.L., Xu, H.X., Pan, X.P., Gao, C.Y., Han, N., Fu, M.Y. "Garlic and gastric cancer" *Acta Nutria Sinica* (4) 53, 1982.

Garlic's natural nitrate scavenging capabilities were also demonstrated by an experiment conducted at the Shandong Medical University in China. Nine volunteers were given 300 mg of nitrates and 500 mg of proline, a proven nitrosamine producing combination. **Blood levels of nitrosamine** were predictably raised after ingestion of the nitrate-proline supplement. But after receiving 5 grams (5,000 mg) of fresh garlic, the nitrate-proline combination failed to produce any detectable increase in blood nitrosamine.

Taking this one step further, another Chinese experiment studied what would happen if **human stomach cancer cells** were exposed to garlic. Tissue cultures of the stomach cancer cells showed that garlic and **diallyl trisulfide** was as effective in inhibiting cancer cell growth as some chemotherapeutic agents.

Pan, X.Y. "Comparison of the cytotoxic effect of fresh garlic, diallyl trisulfide, 5-flurouracil, mitomycin C and cis-DDP on two lines of gastric cancer cells" *Chung-Hua Chung Liu Tsa Chih* (7) 103, 1985.

University of Minnesota at Minneapolis researchers have reported that the administration of **allyl methyl trisulfide**, a garlic oil constituent, reduced the development of **stomach cancer** in mice exposed to benzopyrene by 70 percent.

Sparnins, V.L., Mott, A.W., Barany, G., Wattenberg, L.W. "Effects of allyl methyl trisulfide on glutathione S-transferase activity and benzopyrene-induced neoplasia in the mouse" *Nutrition and Cancer* (8) 211, 1986.

Stomach cancer is not the only neoplasm prevented by garlic's reduction of nitrosoamines. In the recent February 1994 issue of *Carcinogenesis*, Lin, Liu, and Milner reported the ability of garlic powder to protect against carcinogen production in **rat breast** tissue.

Lin, X.Y., Liu, J.Z., Milner, J.A. "Dietary garlic suppresses DNA adducts caused by N-nitroso compounds" *Carcinogenesis* (1994 Feb) 15(2):349–52

Aflatoxin, that sinister peanut fungus carcinogen, can stimulate the production of kidney and liver tumors in 20% of the *Bufo regularis* toad population. But when fresh minced garlic and garlic oil is added to their diet, all but only 3% of these amphibians can resist the aflatoxin cancers.

el-Mofty, M.M., Sakr, S.A. Essawy, A., Abdel Gawad, H.S. "Preventive action of garlic on aflatoxin B1-induced carcinogenesis in the toad Bufo regularis" *Nutr Cancer* (1994) 21(1):95–100

Radiation Protection

Ionizing radiation is a recognized cause of cancer. Epidemiological studies have shown a direct cause and effect relationship between the exposure to radiation experienced by X-ray technicians, radiologists, dentists, uranium miners, and survivors of nuclear bombings with very high incidents of cancer.

Research at the M.D. Anderson Cancer Center in Houston looked at the **protection** garlic offers during exposure **to radiation**. Mice exposed to high level gamma ray radiation show clear evidence of colon cellular damage that frequently leads to cancer. But the administration of *diallyl sulfide* (DAS), present in garlic, before radiation exposure significantly inhibited cellular mutations.

A study of women undergoing radiotherapy and chemotherapy for gynecological malignancies was conducted in Japan. One group took 2 capsules (2 ml) of Kyolic aged garlic extract a day for one to nine months. A second control group took a placebo. Most of those taking the garlic (67%) reported no side effects at all while taking their cancer treatments, and the remainder reported significantly fewer and less severe side effects.

> Tanaka, M. "Clinical studies of Kyoleopin on complaints following treatment of gynecological malignancies" *Japanese Journal of New Remedies* (31) 1349, 1982.

Benjamin Lau investigated the **radiation protection** effects of garlic compounds on **human lymphocytes** in tissue culture. Several lymphocyte cultures were incubated with Kyolic, fresh garlic extract (using 2.5 mg/ml concentrations) and L-cysteine (at 1 mg/ml), as well as a control incubated alone. Then one of each test culture was reserved for continued incubation and one was irradiated with 2000 rads from a Linear Accelerator. The cells in all cultures were tested for viability at 3, 12, 24, 48, and 72 hours. The results are shown in figure 6.

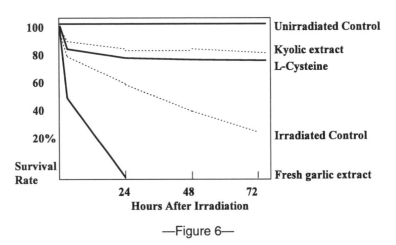

—Figure 6—

Australian scientists at the University of Sydney studied the effects of garlic in preventing **skin cancer**. Garlic was found to provide significant protection against harmful solar ultraviolet rays. Garlic-fed mice developed 58 percent fewer skin cancer cells than mice on a garlic-free diet.

Another consequence of sunbathing is a suppression of the body's immune system. Garlic to the rescue again! Further confirmation of garlic's protection against the Sun's damaging UV rays was reported in the December 1993 issue of *Photochemistry and Photobiology*. This time lyophilized aged garlic extract was fed to hairless mice and observed for any reduction in the immunosuppressive effects of UV radiation. Garlic suppressed the suppression by nearly 60 percent!

Reeve, V.E., Bosnic, M., Rozinova, E., Boehm-Wilcox, C. "A garlic extract protects from ultraviolet B (280–320 nm) radiation-induced suppression of contact hypersensitivity" *Photochem Photobiol* (1993 Dec) 58(6):813–7

The College of Pharmacy at Dakota State University studied the effects of directly applying garlic compounds to the skin of mice. **Diallyl sulfide** and **diallyl disulfide**, present in garlic, was applied to test mice who were exposed to **UV radiation**. There was a significant increase in the survival of mice treated with the garlic compounds.

Pretreating cancer-free mice at Kansas State University with **dipropenyl sulfide**, another important compound found in garlic, produced 86 percent fewer tumors than untreated mice after exposure to **topical carcinogenic** chemicals. "These results indicate that garlic oil inhibits all stages of mouse skin tumorigenesis," they concluded.

Breast cancer cell growth is also inhibited by garlic. S.G. Sundaram, et al, wanted to see what differences there might be between the water-soluble and oil-soluble organic sulfur compounds extracted from garlic. They studied canine tumor cells in culture taken from dogs with induced breast cancers. Only the **oil-soluble** derivatives (**diallyl sulfide**-disulfide-trisulfide) produced marked inhibition of neoplastic cell growth.

Sundaram, S.G., Milner, J.A. "Impact of organosulfur compounds in garlic on canine mammary tumor cells in culture" *Cancer Lett* (1993 Oct 15) 74(1–2):85–90

Sidney Belman at the New York University Medical Center studied the development of **skin cancer** in mice exposed to dimethyl benzanthracene. Once again, topical garlic oil applications prevented tumor formation.

Belman, S. "Onion and garlic oils inhibit tumor promotion" *Carcinogenesis* (4) 1063, 1983.

Dr. Michael J. Wargovich, associate professor of medicine at the University of Texas's M.D. Anderson Cancer Center, reported that **organic sulfides, like diallyl sulfide** found in garlic, prevent the development of **esophageal** and **colon cancer** induced in rodents by the potent carcinogen dimethyl hydrazine. Wargovich believes garlic is "a promising cancer chemopreventitive" for humans as well.

Wargovich, M.J., Goldberg, M.T. "Diallyl sulfide: a naturally occurring thioether that inhibits carcinogen-induced nuclear damage to colon epithelial cells in vivo" *Mutation Research* (143) 127, 1985.
Wargovich, M.J. "Diallyl sulfide, a flavor component of garlic (Allium sativum), inhibits dimethylhydrazine-induced colon cancer" *Carcinogenesis* (8) 487, 1987.

Wargovich got his lead 10 years ago from the work of Eric Block at Albany's New York State University. He tried garlic oil in his mouse gut cancer experiments and saw some tumor suppression. What was it in garlic oil that was causing the cancer inhibition? With varying reports of from 60 to 100 different chemical ingredients, he was relieved to discover that the food industry had already isolated dozens of the mysterious components. His lab ordered a dozen and began testing them.

In short order he soon identified "an extremely active substance" that "to this day is one of the most powerful anticarcinogens around." **Diallyl sulfide** (DAS) inhibits the formation of mouse tumors in the colon that have been induced by 1,2-dimethylhydrazine (DMH). Furthermore, Wargovich discovered that tumor inhibition correlated in direct proportion to the dose of DAS. Diallyl sulfide also proved to *completely* inhibit tumors from developing in the esophagi of mice (induced with nitrosomethylbenzylamine, NMBA) if it was administered *before* the NMBA.

A very encouraging plus for DAS is the fact that it doesn't appear to have any adverse tumorogenesis side-effects. Many other promising agents that have successfully blocked the early phases of cancer development in one organ were discarded for use in humans because the same drug would cause tumors to sprout up somewhere else after long-term testing.

One obvious disadvantage of using DAS as the ideal food-friendly chemopreventitive is that it reeks right up there with a good many other sulfur-related favorites. Another problem is its oil solubility, a property that makes it vulnerable to damage from heat. Cooking garlic kills a lot of its cancer preventing DAS.

Investigations of some of garlic's water-soluble molecules may reveal an effective yet palatable component. One such is **S-allyl-cysteine** (SAC). Though not quite as effective (SAC requires *larger doses* than DAS *for tumor inhibition)*, it *is* less toxic.

There is growing evidence that the liver plays a crucial role in preventing the development of cancer. Every day our systems are exposed to a variety of environmental carcinogenic substances. Some cancers get a toe hold when the liver, while innocently trying to break down the chemical, unwittingly metabolizes the culprit into an activated form of the carcinogen. The liver's **cytochrome P450** enzyme system is the most common example of this method. DAS is known to inhibit the P450 enzymes and thus prevent activation.

Other cancers take over because they overpower the liver's second line of defense: **detoxification**. A common method of eliminating toxins and potential carcinogens is to remove them from the system by piggybacking them onto a suitable carrier. Glutathione is used in this capacity with the aid of an important enzyme, **glutathione S-transferase**. The resulting complex bundle of molecules are then excreted in the bile. DAS enhances the activity of GS-transferase.

Some investigators have expressed concern that as garlic increases the detoxification activity in the liver, medications and other drugs like analgesics will be excreted right along with the carcinogens. The liver doesn't play any favorites and treats all foreign substances the same, be they drugs or poisons.

In fact, pharmacology appreciates this fact: drugs *are* poisons when administered at doses greater than the recommended therapeutic dose. The problem is that the therapeutic dose is very close to that of the poisonous dose in many instances. Digitalis and theophyllin are two common examples of Jekyl-and-Hyde drugs.

No single food will prevent every kind of cancer in every individual. People are different; cancers are different and the carcinogens that cause them vary. The possibility for success is much more likely when multiple chemopreventive agents are incorporated in a mixed diet including fresh fruits and fresh vegetables. This concept has been confirmed experimentally using combinations of garlic and citrus fruits.

Many kinds of cancer are either directly caused or secondarily activated by various environment and lifestyle factors. Because of this, the search is on for new cancer-preventing compounds that are already present in an edible, palatable food and whose concentrations can be optimized by the same selective breeding techniques that have brought us seedless grapes and burpless cucumbers.

The Holy Grail of such efforts is the ultimate development of effective chemopreventives that can one day be available right off the grocery shelf. In this regard, Wargovich is teaming up with Dr. Leonard Pike, head of the Vegetable Improvement Center at Texas A&M to create the ultimate "designer food."

Pike spent 10 years breeding sulfur compounds out of onions, and produced the popular Texas 1015 supersweet onion. Now he's trying to develop a garlicky-tasting onion that is rich in chemopreventive agents.

Wargovich notes, "In this country, we're a little behind in using foods and herbs for medication."

Dr. Wargovich, Department of Gastrointestinal Medical Oncology and Digestive Diseases, Box 78, The University of Texas M. D. Anderson Cancer Center, 1515 Holcombe Boulevard, Houston, Texas 77030, or call (713) 792–7493.

Patterson, Sunita, *M. D. Anderson Oncology* (39) 1, 1994.

Ajoene, not only is a potent anti-platelet, anti-clotting antibiotic, it has also been shown to have impressive cytotoxic properties against cancer cells. A report by K. Scharfenberg in the January, 1994 issue of *Journal of Cell Physiology* determined the mechanism ajoene uses to produce its lethal effect on tumor cells. Using a **lymphoma**

cell culture they found that ajoene appeared to rapidly oxidize glutathione and cause blisters to form on the cytoplasmic membrane similar to the effects of a thermal or chemical burn. Cancer cells were affected the most because they demonstrated the fastest uptake of ajoene.

Scharfenberg, K., Ryll, T., Wagner, R., Wagner, K.G. "Injuries to cultivated BJA-B cells by ajoene, a garlic-derived natural compound: cell viability, glutathione metabolism, and pools of acidic amino acids" *J Cell Physiol* (1994 Jan) 158(1):55–60

Wart Papiloma Treatment: A Personal Testimony

Nightly application of fresh crushed garlic to a fast-growing varrucous growth achieved complete removal within three days. The garlic "mash," which amounted to $\frac{1}{8}$" diameter piece, was held in place by a small Band-Aid. After the first application, the 2mm pedunculated warty tissue turned white. After the second night, it softened and crumbled. By the third morning, the surrounding skin had turned pink and the stalk separated. A flat scab formed and ultimately flaked off 3 days later.

Longevity

Those prone to longevity appear to prefer garlic over other foods. A study of 8,500 **centenarians** by the National Institute of Aging showed that long-lifers chose garlic and onion as their two most favored foods.

Closely related to longevity are **learning** and **memory performance**. A group of researchers using a special strain of mice published their findings on these important parameters in 1994. These mice, which are a model for Alzheimer-type premature senility in humans, were bred to develop an accelerated form of senescence. When the mice reached the age of 2 months, they were placed on a diet which contained aged garlic extract (AGE) in a concentration of 2%. The treated mice showed a markedly improved ability to not only learn new tasks and acquire new information, but they also retained it longer than the untreated controls. But that's not all. The garlic-fed mice **lived significantly longer** than senile mice without the garlic advantage.

Moriguchi, T., Takashina, K., Chu, P.J., Saito, H., Nishiyama, N. "Prolongation of life span and improved learning in the senescence accelerated mouse produced by aged garlic extract" *Biol Pharm Bull* (1994 Dec) 17(12):1589–94

Rodent benefits are interesting, but what about human studies? Another recent study published in a 1994 issue of the Journal of Ethnopharmacology looked at garlic's anti-aging capabilities on human tissue. They found that cultured human skin fibroblasts exposed to garlic extract were able to repetitively reproduce themselves many more times over that of cells in a standard culture medium. The shape of the cells and the integrity of their intracellular structures was maintained significantly longer than untreated cells. However, these effects were reversed when garlic was added to cancerous fibroblasts. The cancer cells could not survive as many repeated subculturings in the presence of garlic.

> Svendsen, L., Rattan, S.I., Clark, B.F. "Testing garlic for possible anti-ageing effects on long-term growth characteristics, morphology and macromolecular synthesis of human fibroblasts in culture" *J Ethnopharmacol* (1994 Jul 8) 43(2):125–33

Diabetes

Garlic has shown a consistent ability to lower elevated blood sugar levels. It appears to be just what the doctor ordered for those suffering from or with a high risk family history of diabetes mellitus.

The mechanism by which it affects blood sugar appears to be either its ability to stimulate the pancreas to increase insulin production or make protein-bound insulin physiologically available, or positively affect blocked cell membrane insulin-receptors, or some combination of the above. Future research will undoubtedly determine the exact mechanism.

As early as 1958, Indian researchers reported the ability of garlic to reduce elevated blood sugar levels. They gave garlic juice to diabetic rabbits and noted a **rapid reduction** in the rabbits' **blood sugar levels.**

> Jain, R.C., Vyas, C.R., Mahatma, O.P. "Hypoglycaemic Action of Onion and Garlic" *Lancet* (2) 1491, December 19, 1973.

Another *Lancet* article, September 11, 1976, reported the **hypoglycemic effects of garlic** and onion. Up to 4 capsules of Kyolic Garlic or about 7 drops of Great American's green onion-garlic oil is suggested for diabetics on a daily basis.

Similar tests performed on rabbits by researchers at the RNT Medical College in India demonstrated that feeding garlic produced a drop in blood sugar levels **comparable to** that of the diabetic medication **tolbutamine**. They proposed that garlic may act by stimulating pancreatic secretion or releasing bound insulin.

Jain, R.C., Vyas, C.R. "Garlic in alloxan-induced diabetic rabbits" *American Journal of Clinical Nutrition* (28) 684, 1975.

The United States Department of Agriculture published an extensive study of garlic and its influence on carbohydrate metabolism. They showed that feeding garlic to rats caused an **increase** in their **serum insulin levels.**

Chang, M.L, Johnson, M.A. "Effect of Garlic on Carbohydrate Metabolism and Lipid Synthesis in Rats" *Journal of Nutrition* (110) 931, 1980.

Even more impressive was a study performed by the Wakunaga Pharmaceutical company on the ability of liquid Kyolic garlic extract to **prevent a rise in blood sugar levels** that are normally expected after taking the oral loading dose of glucose in a standard glucose tolerance test.

Nagai, K., Nakagawa, S., Nojima, S. Mimori, H. "Effect of aged Garlic Extract on Glucose Tolerance Test in Rats" *Basic Pharmacology and Therapeutics* (3) 45, 1975.

Not only does garlic improve insulin-sugar metabolism in diabetic individuals, but it can also make glucose available in a more efficient manner in normal non-diabetics. This accounts for the many reports of increased endurance and greater energy purported by those who have eaten garlic regularly.

A study of rat swimming times illustrates this phenomena. Groups of rats were fed either garlic oil, garlic juice or saline for a period of seven days. The 'guinea pig' rodents were thrown into a container of water and the clock started. The control rats could dog paddle only 480 seconds before giving up. The rats who had sipped on fresh garlic juice for the previous week could tread water for an additional 36 seconds. But those who had received the aged garlic oil just kept on going—for another 324 seconds! They could swim nearly twice as long as their garlic-deprived cohorts. The results of this study are shown in figure 7.

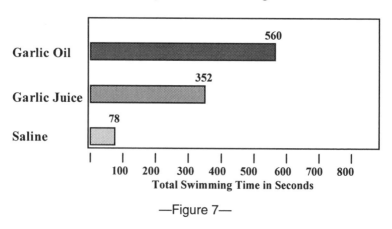

—Figure 7—

Then the researchers injected the same rats with isoproterenol, a drug that induces an artificial state of panic: the heart races several times normal speed and can actually induce heart damage. When the rats were tested this time, there was a dramatic difference between the three groups as shown in figure 8.

Saxena, K.K., Gupta, B., Kulshrestha, V.K., Srivastava, R.K., Prasad, D.N. "effect of garlic pretreatment on isoprenaline-induced myocardial necrosis in albino rats"

Indian Journal of Physiology and Pharmacology (24) 233, 1980.

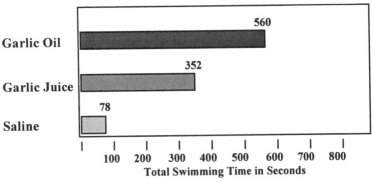

Endurance After Isoproterenol
—Figure 8—

Now the controls petered-out after only 78 seconds, an 84% loss of endurance. But, while the rats in the garlic-groups also suffered, they only dropped by a little over 30%. Garlic was able to protect them from the artificially-induced state of abnormal stress.

Studies in humans also demonstrate that energy and stress seem to be inversely related. Hospitalized patients were evaluated for the energy-related benefits of garlic at Sakitama Hospital in Japan. The patients were divided into two groups. One group took 4 ml of Kyolic aged garlic extract daily for 50 days. The other group served as controls and took a placebo. The garlic supplemented group reported faster recovery from exhaustion, fewer complaints of work-induced fatigue, and less coldness in their extremities than did the group taking the placebo.

Hasegawa, Y., Kikuchi, n., Kawashima, Y., Ono, Y., Shimizu, K., Nishiyama, M. "Clinical effects of Kyoleopin against various complaints in the field of internal medicine" *Japanese Journal of New Remedies* (32) 365, 1983.

Anti-inflammatory Effects

Garlic has been shown to reduce inflammation by inhibiting the enzymes lipoxygenase and cyclooxygenase which are involved in the conversion of arachidonic acid to two different eicosanid pathways. The eicosanids are precursors in the production of various prostaglandins. **Prostaglandins**, originally isolated from semen, were initially thought to be part of the prostate gland secretions. Now they are known to exist in all tissues and are potent mediators of many physiologic processes.

Studying the effects of garlic on cases of lumbago and arthritis, the Department of Surgery at Fukuyama Army Hospital in Japan reported an 86% improvement in patients receiving Kyolic extract.

Garlic's anti-inflammatory properties have made it useful in alleviating the burning and stinging pain of insect and scorpion stings.

Detoxification

Kyolic, the raw garlic extract developed in Japan, effectively protects against **heavy metal poisoning**. Drs. Kitahara, Ikezoe, and Yamada studied both rabbits and humans and reported that garlic prevented erythrocyte (red blood cell) membrane damage from the effects of various heavy metals like lead, mercury, cadmium, arsenic, etc. *Kiso-to-Rinsho,* March, 1975.

V. Petrov recorded the experience of industrial workers in a Russian journal. Daily doses of garlic extract were given to the workers who had been suffering from chronic **lead poisoning**. Symptoms improved and the high urine porphyrin levels dropped. Incidentally, they noted that many of the workers who had a history of hypertension experienced a dramatic normalization of their blood pressure. The article attributed the results to the high concentration of sulfur compounds in garlic.

Petkov, V., Stoev, V., Bakalov, D., Petev L. "The Bulgarian drug Satal as a remedy for lead intoxication in industrial conditions" *Higiena Truda i Profesionalnie Zabolevanya*, (4) 42, 1965.

The ability of garlic to soak up heavy metals was demonstrated again in a 1994 report from Germany. These investigators studied the **lead levels in chickens** who were fed garlic and/or lead acetate. Garlic was able to 'get the lead out' even if given *after* exposure to lead. The authors believe garlic contains an organic chelating compound that could be used to reduce environmental pollution in meat products. More importantly, it works for us humans as well.

> Hanafy, M.S., Shalaby, S.M., el-Fouly, M.A. Abd el-Aziz, M.I., Soliman, F.A. "Effect of garlic on lead contents in chicken tissues" *DTW Dtsch Tierarztl Wochenschr* (1994 Apr) 101(4):157–8

The **heavy metal binding capacity** of garlic was studied by Drs. S. Kitahara, H. Sumiyoshi, and K. Kamiota. Laboratory rats were injected with Methylmercuric chloride intravenously. Fecal analyses were then conducted over the following seven days on two cohorts of seven rats each. Figure 9 illustrates their findings. The group receiving the Japanese garlic extract, Kyolic, eliminated mercury 2–4 times faster than the control group.

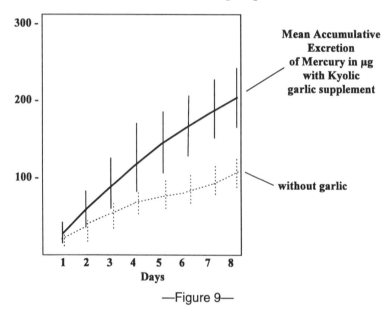

—Figure 9—

The effect of garlic in increasing elimination of heavy metals (CH_3HgCl) in rodents.

More interesting was the finding that garlic has a selective affinity to heavy metals while sparing the biologically important electrolytes such as potassium, magnesium, calcium, and zinc. See figure 10. This property makes garlic a nearly ideal detoxifying agent. Undesirable side-effects are not observed.

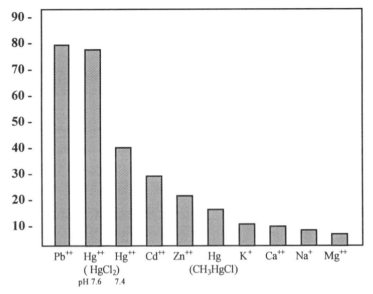

Garlic-enhanced Binding Capacity in mg/g
—Figure 10—

Dr. Tohru Fuwa at the Central Research Laboratories of Wakunaga Pharmaceutical Company in Japan studied the protective effects of garlic on liver cells exposed to toxic chemicals. He observed that liver cells in tissue culture were spared the damaging effects that carbon tetrachloride can cause when certain constituents of garlic are present. Four of the six identified sulfur-containing compounds found in garlic were effective in preventing toxic liver cell damage.

Nakagawa, S., Yoshida, S., Hirao, Y., Kasuga, S., Fuwa, T. "Cytoprotective activity of compounds of Garlic, Ginseng and Ciuwjia on Hepatocyte Injury Induced by Carbon

Tetrachloride In Vitro" *Hiroshima Journal of Medical Science* (34) 303, 1985.

The actual compounds responsible for the protective effect were isolated and identified by Dr. Hiroshi Hikino and his colleagues at the Pharmaceutical Institute of Tohoku University. They determined that two sulfur-containing amino acids, **S-allylmercapto cysteine** (ASSC) and **S-methylcercapto cysteine** (MSSC), could be extracted from garlic and prevent the damage of liver cells when exposed to potent liver toxins like carbon tetrachloride and D-galactosamine. They discovered that these garlic compounds where able to provide such amazing protection by inhibiting the generation of *free radicals* which cause cellular damage by oxidizing lipid peroxides.

Hikino, H., Tohkin, M., Kiso, Y., Namiki, T., Nishimura, S., Takeyama, K. "Antihepatotoxic Actions of Allium sativum Bulbs" *Planta Medica* (3) 163, 1986.

Another study conducted by a group lead by Dr. Kyoichi Kagawa looked at the therapeutic value of garlic on liver damage. In this study, the researchers fed mice the liver damaging carbon tetrachloride. "Carbon tet" (CCl_4) is converted to carbon trichloride (CCl_3) within the liver. It is this compound that attacks unsaturated fatty acids and breaks them down into triglyceride chains. These fatty acid chains then accumulate in the liver causing a pathological condition called "fatty liver." When these same mice were fed garlic extract up to six hours after exposure to the poisonous carbon tetrachloride, they would not develop fatty liver injury.

Kagawa, K., Matsutaka, H., Yamaguchi, Y., Fukuhama, C. "Garlic extract inhibits the enhanced peroxidation and production of lipids in carbon tetrachloride-induced liver injury" *Japanese Journal of Pharmacology* (42) 19, 1986.

Recipes and Formulae

Garlic Syrup

Peel, chop or mince 1 lb. fresh garlic.
Place in wide mouth jar. Add equal parts vinegar and distilled water to just cover the garlic. Close tightly, shake well, and let stand for 4 days, thoroughly shaking once or twice a day. Then add 1 pint of glycerine, shake well and let stand another day. Strain with pressure. Filter liquid through linen cloth. Add 3 lb. pure honey and stir until blended.

For flavor and masking the pungent garlic odor, replace the vinegar and distilled water in the above recipe with the following:

Take 1 quart vinegar, add 3 ounces powdered caraway seed and 3 ounces sweet fennel seed, boil for 15 minutes, closely covered. Strain and when cold add 1 point of glycerin.

Dosage:
For asthma, coughs:
1 tsp every 15 minutes until spasm is controlled followed by 1 tsp every 2–3 hours for the remainder of the day. Then 1 tsp 3–4 times a day.
Tuberculosis, pulmonary edema:
2–3 tsp three to four times a day (between meals).
Children: 8–15 years: half the adult dose.
              5–7 years: one quarter the adult dose.
              1–4 years: one eighth the adult dose.

Topical Garlic Preparations:

For eczema, exanthems, psoriasis, skin ulcers, skin cancer, adenopathy, necrotic wounds, septic wounds.

8 ounces fresh garlic juice
8 ounces glycerin
Mix thoroughly and add 1 pint of burdock seed tea
Directions:
Saturate gauze or cotton swab and apply to affected areas. Cover with an occlusive plastic dressing (Saran Wrap) and bandage.
Change 2–3 times daily. Take oral garlic syrup as well.

Garlic Paste:
Peel and mash one garlic clove and apply to bee stings and other painful or inflamed insect bites.

Garlic Plaster:
Peel and mash several cloves into a paste then spread onto cheesecloth or muslin and fold to close. Apply to skin taking care not to allow the garlic paste to come in direct contact.

Garlic Compress:
Boil water
Peel and chop several cloves, add to boiling water
Steep for 15 minutes
Cool to less than 180 degrees
Soak small soft cloth in the liquid, wring slightly and apply. Cover the wet cloth with a dry towel and leave until warmth is no longer felt. Replace with new warm cloth and repeat until tingling is detected (about 30 minutes).

Ear Aches:
Apply a few drops of warm garlic oil extract to affected ear and seal with a small cotton pledget.
Slice a peeled garlic clove into small chunks.

Add a small quantity of olive oil and heat briefly.
Strain chunks and use garlic oil as above.
Garlic extract oil is also useful as an antiflatulent.
Dose: 1 tsp.

Garlic Bread

> ¼ cup olive oil
> ½ tsp dried oregano
> 1 tsp dried basil
> 4 cloves garlic

1 small loaf whole-grain bread cut in thick slices.
Mix together butter, oregano and basil in a small bowel.
Peel and chop garlic in small pieces and add to mixture.
Refrigerate overnight. Preheat oven to 350°. Spread both
sides of bread with garlic butter, arrange into loaf, and
wrap with aluminum foil. Bake for 20 minutes and serve.

Sour Cream and Garlic Salad Dressing

> 1 cup imitation sour cream
> 2 tsp mustard spread
> 1 tsp honey
> 1½ Tbs lemon juice
> ½ tsp minced garlic

Combine all ingredients and mix well. Refrigerate leftovers
and mix thoroughly before each use.

Tomato-Garlic Pasta Sauce

> 2 lb ripe tomatoes
> ¼ cup olive oil
> 4 cloves chopped garlic
> 2 medium chopped onions
> 1 tsp salt

¼ tsp dried oregano

3 tsp dried basil

2 tsp chopped parsley

Immerse tomatoes in boiling water for 12 seconds. Peel and chop into 1-inch pieces. Heat oil in 10–12 inch skillet over medium heat. Add garlic and onions. Cook, stirring regularly. Add tomatoes, salt, pepper, oregano, basil and parsley when the onions become transparent. Cook uncovered over low heat for 2 hours. Stir occasionally. Makes 4 cups.

Garlic and Oil Pasta Sauce

½ cup olive oil

5 or more whole garlic cloves

1 small dried hot chili pepper

1 Tbs minced fresh parsley

Heat oil slowly in small pan. When hot, add garlic cloves and chili pepper. Cook until garlic is slightly brown. Remove garlic and chili pepper. Remove from heat and allow oil to cool a few minutes. Toss with hot pasta. Add parsley and toss again.

Appendix

Additional Annotated Technical References by Topic

Longevity

Moriguchi, T., Takashina, K., Chu, P.J., Saito, H., Nishiyama, N. "Prolongation of life span and improved learning in the senescence accelerated mouse produced by aged garlic extract" *Biol Pharm Bull* (1994 Dec) 17(12):1589–94

This was a study conducted on a special strain of mice that have been bred to demonstrate premature senility, the senescence accelerated mouse or SAM. The researchers wanted to see what effect **aged garlic extract** (AGE) would have on the **longevity, learning** and **memory** performance of mentally impaired mice. Beginning at the age of 2 months, these mice were fed a diet containing 2% AGE.

The survival ratio of those mice in the P8 strain which were treated with AGE was significantly higher than that of untreated controls. AGE, however, did not affect the life span of a senescence-resistant R1 strain. AGE also did not seem to have any effect on body weight or motor activity. In passive and conditioned avoidance tests, AGE appeared to markedly improve memory acquisition and retention processes in both the SAM P8 and R1 groups. These results suggest that AGE might possibly be useful for the treatment of **physiological aging** and **age-related memory deficits in humans**.

Svendsen, L., Rattan, S.I., Clark, B.F. "Testing garlic for possible anti-ageing effects on long-term growth characteristics, morphology and macromolecular synthesis of human fibroblasts in culture" *J Ethnopharmacol* (1994 Jul 8) 43(2):125–33

In addition to the acknowledged beneficial effects claimed for the use of garlic as a nutritional supplement (which include **detoxification, antioxidation, antifungal activity, antibacterial activity,** and **tumor suppression**) this study considered the possible **anti-aging** and rejuvenating effects that have been promoted. The authors used the **Hayflick system of cellular ageing in culture.** They tested garlic for its anti-aging effects by measuring the long-term growth characteristics, morphology and macromolecular synthesis of **human skin fibroblasts**. Their results showed that an addition of garlic extract into the normal cell culture medium allowed them to perform serial subculturing of the same cell culture for more than 55 population doublings within 475 days. They measured the **anti-aging** effects on the human fibroblasts by measuring their **maximum proliferative capacity** and preserved **morphological characteristics**. They noted paradoxically that similar or even smaller doses of garlic extracts exhibited a **growth inhibitory effect on cancerous cells.** They also observed that cancerous cells could not be grown over these longer periods of time in the presence of garlic.

Antibiotic Effects

Pai, S.T., Platt, M.W. "Antifungal effects of Allium sativum (garlic) extract against the Aspergillus species involved in otomycosis" *Lett Appl Microbiol* (1995 Jan) 20(1):14–8

Otomycosis (external ear canal linfections due to saprophytic keratolytic fungi) represents a relative small percentage of all clinical **external otitis cases.** Garlic is currently utilized as a folk medicine in many countries for its antimicrobial and other beneficial properties. In response to a lack of effective otic preparations, the authors of this study set out to see just how effective garlic extracts would be against the fungi belonging to the genus **Aspergillus.** They included in their study two garlic preparations: **Aqueous garlic extract (AGE)** and **concentrated garlic oil (CGO).** In addition they included various commercial garlic supplements and pharmaceutical prescriptions indicated for the treatment of fungal otic infections were used in an in-vitro study. AGE and **especially CGO were found to have antifungal activity.** which demonstrated **similar or better inhibitory effects than the pharmaceutical preparations** and exhibited **similar minimum inhibitory concentrations.**

Guo, N.L., Lu, D.P., Woods, G.L., Reed, E., Zhou, G.Z., Zhang, L.B., Waldman, R.H. "Demonstration of the anti-viral activity of garlic extract against human cytomegalovirus in vitro" *Chin Med J* (Engl) (1993 Feb) 106(2):93–6

The **anti-viral activity of garlic extract** (GE) on **human cytomegalovirus (HCMV) was evaluated by studying the reduction in viral plaque size and early antigen levels on in vitro tissue culture.** When garlic extract was applied simultaneously with HCMV an **inhibition of the virus** was measured that was directly proportional to the GE dose. But the effect was stronger when the tissue culture monolayers were pretreated with GE. In addition, the **anti-viral effect of garlic persisted in infected cells long after it was removed from the culture medium.** The strongest anti-viral effect of GE was demonstrated when it was continuously applied to the cells. The researchers recommended that when garlic is used clinically for the treatment of HCMV infection it should be delivered in a persistent manner and that the **use of Garlic Extract for the prophylaxis of HCMV is preferable over treatment of the active infection in immunocompromised patients**.

> Urbina, J.A., Marchan, E., Lazardi, K., Visbal, G., Apitz-Castro, R., Gil, F., Aguirre, T., Piras, M.M., Piras, R. "Inhibition of phosphatidylcholine biosynthesis and cell proliferation in Trypanosoma cruzi by ajoene, an antiplatelet compound isolated from garlic" *Biochem Pharmacol* (1993 Jun 22) 45(12):2381-7

Ajoene (technically referenced as **(E,Z)-4,5,9-trithiadodeca-1,6,11-triene 9-oxide**), is a **potent antiplatelet compound** derived from garlic. This study demonstrated its ability to **inhibit** the proliferation of both epimastigote and amastigote stages in the life cycle of **Trypanosoma cruzi**, the protazoal organism which causes **Chagas' disease**. The growth of the epimastigote form was observed to be **immediately arrested** by only **80 microM of ajoene**, and **100 microM induced cell lysis** (caused the cells to rupture) **within 24 hr.** In the amastigote form proliferating inside live cells, only **40 microM of ajoene** was needed to completely **eradicate the parasite** from the host cells in 96 hr. This study also determined that the inhibition by ajoene of the growing epimastigotes caused by ajoene took place at the same time that they noticed a major change in the phospholipid composition of the treated cells. Phosphatidylcholine (PC), the major phospholipid present in control cells, dropped to unusually low levels, while its immediate precursor, phosphatidylethanolamine (PE), became dominant. The fatty acids which were esterified in this lipid fraction underwent a dramatic change due to the increase in the content of saturated fatty acids and a **marked reduction in the content of linoleic (18:2) acid.** Linoleic acid was the predominant fatty acid in control cells. The researchers also found that **ajoene inhibited the de novo synthesis** (from scratch) **of neutral lipids**

and, in particular, of **sterols** in the epimastigotes, but the resultant changes in the sterol composition were not sufficient to explain the antiproliferative effects of the drug. So they used an **electron-microscopy** and saw a **concentration-dependent alteration** of intracellular membranous structures, particularly the **mitochondrion** and **endoplasmatic reticulum**. These results suggest that the antiproliferative effects of ajoene against *Trapanosoma cruzi* is closely related to its **specific alteration of the cell's phospholipid composition**.

> Davis, L.E., Shen, J., Royer, R.E. "In vitro synergism of concentrated *Allium sativum* extract and amphotericin B against Cryptococcus neoformans" *Planta Med* (1994 Dec) 60(6):546–9

This study wanted to evaluate the scientific merit of using allicin-derived compounds as an anti-fungal drug. So they looked at the use of garlic both alone and with amphotericin B for the treatment of **human systemic fungal infections** and **cryptococcal meningitis**. They prepared a concentrated garlic extract that contained **34% allicin, 44% total thiosulfinates**, and **20% vinyldithiins**. When this form of garlic was used they found that the concentrated extract possessed **potent in vitro fungistatic and fungicidal activity** against 3 different isolates of **Cryptococcus neoformans**. The *minimum inhibitory concentration* of the concentrated garlic extract against 100,000 organisms of *C. neoformans* ranged from *6 to 12 micrograms/ml*. In addition, the authors noticed that there was a significant **in vitro synergistic fungistatic activity with amphotericin B** which was demonstrated against all of the *C. neoformans* isolates. In other words, the effectiveness of garlic or amphotericin B when used alone in killing fungal organisms was enhanced in more than simply an additive way when both garlic *and* amphotericin B were used together. The study provides objective laboratory support for the treatment of cryptococcal infections with concentrated garlic extracts.

> Gonzalez-Fandos, E., Garcia-Lopez, M.L., Sierra, M.L., Otero, A. "Staphylococcal growth and enterotoxins (A-D) and thermonuclease synthesis in the presence of dehydrated garlic" *J Appl Bacteriol* (1994 Nov) 77(5):549–52

This study looked at how garlic inhibited the growth of **Staphylococcus aureus** and the production of its enterotoxin and thermonuclease in a culture of BHI broth. The growth of Staph. aureus was inhibited by **dehydrated garlic** at levels equal to or greater than 1.5% (w/v). **Enterotoxins A, B and C1** became undetectable once the concentration of garlic in the broth reached or exceeded 1%. **Enterotoxin D** was produced up to a level of 2%. The researchers also noted that garlic **inhibited thermonuclease (TNAse)** production at garlic concentrations or = 1.5%.

Sulfur Compounds

> Calvey, E.M., Roach, J.A., Block, E. "Supercritical fluid chromatography of garlic (Allium sativum) extracts with mass spectrometric identification of allicin" [published erratum appears in *J Chromatogr Sci* 1994 Sep;32(9):4A] *J Chromatogr Sci* (1994 Mar) 32(3):93–6

This paper describes the author's use of **supercritical fluid chromatography-mass spectrometry** to successfully identify **allicin** (which is formally described in biochemical terms as **2-propene-1-sulfinothioic acid S-2-propenyl ester**). Allicin is *the predominant thiosulfinate in freshly cut garlic*. The rest of the article is of a very technical nature dealing with the effects of the restrictor tip and oven temperatures on their ability to obtain a **chemi-**

cal ionization mass spectrum of allicin with "the protonated molecular ion, m/z 163, as the major ion." See what I mean?

> Slepko, G.I., Lobareva, L.S., Mikhalenko, L.Ia., Shatniuk, L.N. "[Biologically active garlic compounds and perspectives of their use in the therapeutic and prophylactic diet (review)] Biologicheski aktivnye komponenty chesnoka i perspektivy ikh ispolzovaniia v lechebno-profilakticheskom pitanii (obzor)" *Vopr Pitan* (1994) (5):28–32

This article reviews the various therapeutic actions of garlic and garlic preparations on vascular and cardiac diseases, digestive organs, lipid exchange and systemic mycosis. The authors noted that beneficial effects in each of these diverse conditions were connected with the presence of various complex sulfur-containing compounds, such as: **thiosulfinates, dialkilsulfides, dithiins, adgoens,** and **thioglycosidepeptides**. These compounds were either isolated from garlic or synthesized to a compound that would render a corresponding physiologic action in an organism. They concluded that garlic preparations (as a component of nutrition) can be effective for use in prophylactic nutrition and diet therapy affecting various body systems.

> Biedermann, B. "[Garlic—a 'secret miracle of God'"?] Knoblauch—ein 'geheimstes Wunder Gottes'?" *Schweiz Rundsch Med Prax* (1995 Jan 3) 84(1):7–10

This paper (written in German) summarizes a number of clinical studies on the effects and side effects of garlic consumption. Antitumor and antiarteriosclerotic effects were demonstrated in vitro and supported by epidemiologic studies. The authors commented that the production of commercial products and pharmacologic studies are handicapped by chemical instability and the low bioavailability of the active compounds.

Ohsumi, C., Hayashi, T. "The oligosaccharide units of the xyloglucans in the cell walls of bulbs of onion, garlic and their hybrid" *Plant Cell Physiol* (1994 Sep) 35(6):963–7

This is a fairly esoteric paper on some rather detailed biochemical aspects of garlic and onion constituents in the carbohydrate realm.

Xyloglucans were isolated by the authors from a 24% KOH-soluble fraction of the cell walls of onion and garlic bulbs and their hybrid. The **polysaccharides** turned out to have average molecular weights of 65,000 for onion, 55,000 for garlic and 82,000 for the hybrid. Compositional analysis of the oligosaccharide units indicated that the polysaccharides were **constructed of four kinds of repeating oligosaccharide units**, namely a:

decasaccharide (glucose/xylose/galactose/fucose, 4 : 3: 2 : 1)
nonasaccharide (glucose/xylose/galactose/fucose, 4 : 3 : 1 : 1)
octasaccharide (glucose/xylose/galactose, 4 : 3 : 1), and a
heptasaccharide (glucose/xylose, 4 : 3).

The xyloglucan from the hybrid contained highly fucosylated units that resembled those from onion rather than from garlic. The analysis also revealed that the xyloglucans from *Allium* species contain **highly substituted xylosyl** and **fucosyl-galactosyl residues**, suggesting that these **monocotyledonous plants resemble dicotyledons** in the structural features of their xyloglucans.

Rabinkov, A., Zhu, X.Z., Grafi, G., Galili, G., Mirelman, D. "Alliin lyase (Alliinase) from garlic (Allium sativum). Biochemical characterization and cDNA cloning" *Appl Biochem Biotechnol* (1994 Sep) 48(3):149–71

Alliinase (EC 4.4.1.4), which **catalyzes the synthesis of allicin**, was purified by the authors of this paper to a high degree of homogeneity from garlic bulbs using various steps, including hydrophobic chromatography. Molecular and biochemical studies showed that the enzyme is **a dimer of two subunits**. The enzyme is **a glycoprotein** containing 6% carbohydrate. Northern and Western blot analyses showed that the bulb alliinase was highly expressed in bulbs, whereas a lower expression level was found in leaves, and no expression was detected in roots. Strikingly, the **roots exhibited an abundant alliinase activity,** suggesting that this tissue expressed **a distinct alliinase isozyme** with **very low homology** to the bulb enzyme ie, it was structurally unrelated.

Nagae, S., Ushijima, M., Hatono, S., Imai, J., Kasuga, S., Matsuura, H., Itakura, Y., Higashi, Y. "Pharmacokinetics of the garlic compound S-allylcysteine" **Planta Med** (1994 Jun) 60(3):214–7

The pharmacokinetic behavior of **S-allylcysteine (SAC),** one of the **biologically active transformation products** from garlic, was investigated by this team of Japanese investigators after its oral administration to **rats, mice, and dogs**. SAC was **rapidly and easily absorbed** in the gastrointestinal tract and distributed mainly in **plasma, liver, and kidney**. The bioavailability was 98.2, 103.0, and 87.2% in rats, mice, and dogs, respectively. SAC was **mainly excreted into the urine** in the N-acetyl form in rats; however, mice excreted both SAC and the N-acetyl form. The half-life of SAC was longer in dogs than in rats and mice.

Vasodilatation and Antihyertensive

Ozturk, Y., Aydin, S., Kosar, M., Baser, K.H. "Endothelium-dependent and independent effects of garlic on rat aorta." *J Ethnopharmacol* (1994 Oct) 44(2):109–16

Effects of garlic in causing relaxation in **isolated rat aorta** were investigated by comparing concentration-response curves obtained from the application of **acetyl-choline, L-arginine** and **garlic**. Garlic (and acetylcholine) caused **dose-dependent relaxations** in isolated rat aorta which were attenuated (but not completely abolished) by the removal of the aortic endothelium. These findings strongly suggested that **the vasorelaxant effect of garlic is important in its hypotensive activity** and is mediated by the production of endothelium-and/or muscle-derived relaxation factors.

Silagy, C.A., Neil, H.A. "A meta-analysis of the effect of garlic on blood pressure" *J Hypertens* (1994 Apr) 12(4):463–8

This was a review article that included a meta-analysis of published and unpublished randomized controlled trials of garlic preparations used to control hypertension. The goal was to determine the effect of **garlic** on **blood pressures** relative to a **placebo** and other **antihypertensive agents**. Studies were identified by a search of two popular electronic databases, from references listed in primary and review articles, and through direct contact with garlic manufacturers. Only randomized controlled trials of garlic preparations were included in the review. And these were required to have lasted at least 4 weeks in duration. Eight trials were identified (all using the same **dried garlic powder preparation (Kwai)** with data from **415 subjects** included in the analyses. Only three of the trials were specifically conducted in hypertensive subjects, and many had other methodological shortcomings. **Of the seven trials** that compared the effect of garlic with that of placebo, **three showed a significant reduction in systolic blood pressure** (SBP) and **four in diastolic** blood pressure (DBP). The **overall pooled mean difference in the absolute change (from baseline to final measurement)** of SBP was greater in the subjects who were treated with garlic then in those treated with placebo. For DBP the correspond-ing reduction in the garlic-treated subjects was slightly smaller. The authors concluded that these results suggest that garlic powder preparation **may be of some clinical use in subjects with mild hypertension**. However, they felt that there was still **insufficient evidence** to recommend it as a **routine clinical therapy** for the treatment of hyper-tensive subjects. More-rigorously designed and analyzed trials are needed.

Estrada, C.A., Young, M.J. "Patient preferences for novel therapy: an N-of-1 trial of garlic in the treatment for hypertension" *J Gen Intern Med* (1993 Nov) 8(11):619–21

The authors used the N-of-1 clinical trial methodology to obtain insights about a **patient's preference for garlic** for the management

of his **hypertension**. The 61-year-old man received garlic, **500 mg by mouth three times a day (for 3 weeks),** or identical placebo (also 3 weeks) in three treatment pairs. While the patient was taking garlic the mean **systolic** blood pressure **decreased by 2 mm Hg** (95% confidence interval 0.4 to 4.7, p 0.05), and the **diastolic** blood pressure de-creased by **2.4 mm Hg** (95% confidence interval 0.4 to 4, p 0.025). The treatment **effect of garlic was small**, but the patient believed continuing garlic for the management of his hypertension was still justified.

McMahon, F.G., Vargas, R. "Can garlic lower blood pressure? A pilot study" *Pharmacotherapy* (1993 Jul-Aug) 13(4):406–7

A popular garlic preparation containing **1.3% allicin at** a large dose **(2400 mg)** was evaluated in this open-label study in **nine patients** with rather **severe hypertension** (**diastolic** blood pressure or = **115 mm Hg**). **Sitting blood pressure fell** $7/16$ (+/- $3/2$ SD) mm Hg at **peak effect** approximately **5 hours after the dose**, with a significant decrease in diastolic blood pressure (p 0.05) from 5–14 hours after the dose. **No significant side effects** were reported. The results of this study indicate that at least *this* garlic preparation can reduce blood pressure. Further controlled studies were recommended, particularly with more conventional doses (e.g., or = 900 mg/day), in patients with mild to moderate hypertension and under placebo-controlled, double-blind conditions.

Cancer Prevention

Amagase, H., Milner, J.A. "Impact of various sources of garlic and their constituents on 7,12-dimethylbenz[a]anthracene binding to mammary cell DNA" *Carcinogenesis* (1993 Aug) 14(8):1627–31

This paper describes a series of studies which were designed to assess the impact of various sources of garlic and their constituents (**water- and ethanol-extracts and S-allylcysteine**) on the **in vivo binding** of a known carcinogen (7,12-dimethylbenz[a]anthracene **DMBA) to rat mammary cell DNA**. It is desirable to keep DNA clean and unaffected by any chemical reaction that could potentially alter its integrity. A molecule can become carcinogenic when it manifests the ability to attach itself to DNA in such a way that the code sequence is altered. One way that garlic demonstrates anticancer properties is in its ability to prevent carcinogens from binding to DNA. In this study the provision of dietary **raw garlic powder (2%) or its water-extract (1.5%) reduced DMBA-DNA binding by 33 and 46% respectively**. Dietary supplementation with a commercially available deodorized garlic powder (powder A) **at 2 or 4%** depressed the occurrence of adducts (carcinogen molecules chemically bound to DNA) **by 50 and 78%** respectively, while providing a commercially available high sulfur garlic preparation (powder B) at 2% reduced binding by 56%. These values represent a very impressive chemoprotective effect of garlic. A pair-feeding study further revealed that the depression in carcinogen binding was independent of food intake or weight gain. Although **1% raw garlic powder did not significantly influence** the occurrence of DMBA-DNA adducts, an equivalent as the **water-extract** (0.75%), the **ethanol-extract** (0.015%) or commercially available **powders (A and B)** reduced DMBA adducts in mammary tissue by **44, 25, 71 and 65%** respectively. **Dietary fortification with S-allylcysteine (SAC), a water-soluble constituent of processed garlic, caused a progressive decrease in the binding of DMBA to DNA.** Studies with SAC **suggest the primary effect of garlic** and its constituents **is on the bioactivation and binding of the carcinogen** rather than DNA repair. These data reveal that several forms of garlic are effective, although variable, in altering carcinogen bioactivation and presumably chemically induced carcinogenesis.

> Sundaram, S.G., Milner, J.A. "Impact of organosulfur compounds in garlic on canine mammary tumor cells in culture" *Cancer Lett* (1993 Oct 15) 74(1–2):85–90

In this study, six organosulfur compounds found in garlic were examined for their ability to alter the growth of **canine mammary tumor cells** (CMT-13) in culture. Three **water-soluble organosulfur compounds (S-allylcysteine, S-ethyl-cysteine and S-propyl-cysteine) did not significantly alter the growth** of CMT-13 cells when added to the cultures at concentrations of 1.0 mM (nanomole) or less. However, three **oil-soluble organosulfur compounds (diallyl sulfide, diallyl disulfide and diallyl trisulfide) markedly inhibited growth**. Increasing addition of diallyl disulfide (DADS) resulted in a progressive decrease in CMT-13 cell growth. **Addition of glutathione before DADS markedly decreased the intensity of the growth inhibition.** Treatment with DL-buthionine-SR-sulfoxamine, a specific inhibitor of glutathione synthesis, accentuated the growth inhibition caused by DADS. These studies show that **some organosulfur compounds found in garlic are effective inhibitors of the growth of the neoplastic CMT-13 cell.** The inhibitory effects of these compounds are modified by intracellular glutathione.

Scharfenberg, K., Ryll, T., Wagner, R., Wagner, K.G. "Injuries to cultivated BJA-B cells by ajoene, a garlic-derived natural compound: cell viability, glutathione metabolism, and pools of acidic amino acids" *J Cell Physiol* (1994 Jan) 158(1):55–60

Ajoene (4,5,9-trithiadodeca-1,6,11-triene-9-oxide), a garlic-derived natural compound, which had been shown to have **cytostatic/cytotoxic properties**, was tested with a **B cell lymphoma-derived cell line** (BJA-B cells) in order to determine the mechanism it uses to produce this cytotoxic action. Viability of the lymphoma cells was determined by the **Trypan blue exclusion test** and the **colorimetric tetrazolium (MTT) assay.** Metabolic disturbances were evaluated by measuring the pools of **reduced (GSH), oxidized glutathione (GSSG)** and the **acidic amino acids, Glu and Asp.** When **ajoene** was added to the cell cultures it was observed to be taken up by the lymphoma cells at a very rapid rate. At the same time there was an **immediate reduction of the GSH** and **increase in the GSSG levels.** The extent of these changes depended on the ajoene dose per cell. At a sublethal ajoene dose the GSH and GSSG pools rose at the later stages to levels much higher than in the control experiment. Bleb formation at the cytoplasmic membrane was a further phenomenon that occurred rapidly, although injuries detected by Trypan blue exclusion developed only at a later stage. The MTT assay, performed in a parallel experiment (48 h after ajoene addition), showed, however, that **reduction of cell viability was established at the very beginning of ajoene exposure**. The action of ajoene strongly resembled **oxidative stress** because of its interference with SH homeostasis and its pleiotropic effects on cell physiology and metabolism.

Das, T., Roychoudhury, A., Sharma, A., Talukder, G. "Modification of clastogenicity of three known clastogens by garlic extract in mice in vivo" *Environ Mol Mutagen* (1993) 21(4):383–8

This study measured the **anticlastogenic activity** of crude garlic extract in the **bone marrow cells of mice**. Male laboratory-bred Swiss albino mice were given one of three concentrations of the **freshly prepared extract (100 mg, 50 mg, and 25 mg/kg body weight) as a dietary supplement by gavage for 6 consecutive days**. On the **seventh day** the mice were administered a single acute dose of two known **clastogens,** either **a combination of mitomycin C(1.5 mg/kg) and cyclophosphamide (25 mg/kg) or sodium arsenite (2.5 mg/kg),** simultaneously with the garlic extract. **After 24 hr**, chromosome preparations were made from the bone marrow cells and inspected for the presence of any **chromosomal aberrations and damaged cells**. Garlic extract alone appeared to induce a low level of chromosomal damage. The **clastogenicity of all three mutagens were reduced significantly in the animals which had been given garlic extract** as a dietary supplement. The extent of this reduction was different for the three clastogens and was thought to be attributed to the interaction with the different components of the extract.

Gao, Y.M., Xie, J.Y., Piao, Y.J. "[Ultrastructural observation of intratumoral neutrophils and macrophages induced by garlic oil]" *Chung Kuo Chung Hsi I Chieh Ho Tsa Chih* (1993 Sep) 13(9):546–8, 518

After **injection of garlic oil in a tumor** focus a large amount of **neutrophils, macrophages and lymphocytes appeared**. Some neutrophils and macrophages were located adjacent to the tumor cells, some of the neutrophils and macrophages penetrated into the intracellular body of the tumor cells. This result showed that **garlic oil could induce neutrophils and macrophages against tumor**.

Lin, X.Y., Liu, J.Z., Milner, J.A. "Dietary garlic suppresses DNA adducts caused by N-nitroso compounds" *Carcinogenesis* (1994 Feb) 15(2):349–52

This study examined the impact of a **processed garlic powder** on the in vivo occurrence of DNA adducts (chemicals that attach themselves to the DNA). Specific DNA adducts, **N-nitroso compounds (NOC),** were created by feeding rats on a diet that contains **aminopyrine** and **sodium nitrite** (at a dose of 600 mg/kg each). When their diet was supplemented with **2% garlic powder the occurrence** of both **7-N-methyldeoxyguanosine** (7-N-mG) and **6-O-methyldeoxyguanosine** (6-O-mG) **adducts to rat liver DNA were reduced** by approximately **55%; and over 80% when 4% garlic** was provided. Dietary supplementation with garlic powder (2 and 4%) also reduced the occurrence of 7-N-mG and 6-O-mG adducts by approximately 40 and 60% respectively, in rats intubated with N-nitrosodimethylamine (150 mg/kg body wt). The quantity of 7-N-mG and 6-O-mG adducts **in mammary tissue** of rats given intravenous N-methyl-N-nitrosourea (50 mg/kg body wt) was **reduced over 50%** in rats fed **2%** garlic compared to controls. The depression in the occurrence of these adducts was approximately **70%** when dietary garlic was increased to **4%.** These experiments suggest the reduction in DNA adducts caused by processed garlic powder likely reflects a **depression in** the formation of

NOC from precursors and changes in the bioactivation and/or denitrosation of NOC.

Reeve, V.E., Bosnic, M., Rozinova, E., Boehm-Wilcox, C. "A garlic extract protects from ultraviolet B (280–320 nm) radiation-induced suppression of contact hypersensitivity" *Photochem Photobiol* (1993 Dec) 58(6):813–7

Lyophilized aged garlic extract has been incorporated at concentrations of **0.1%, 1% and 4% by weight** into a semipurified powdered diet and **fed to hairless mice.** Under **moderate UVB exposure** conditions resulting in 58% **suppression of the systemic contact hypersensitivity response** in control-fed mice, **a dose-responsive protection** was observed in the garlic-fed mice; contact hypersensitivity in the UVB-exposed mice fed 4% garlic extract was suppressed by only 19%. If the UVB exposure was replaced by topical application of one of a series of **lotions** containing increasing concentrations of **cis-urocanic acid**, a dose-responsive **suppression** of **contact hypersensitivity** was demonstrated in control-fed mice (urocanic acid at 25, 50, 100 and 200 micrograms per mouse resulting in 22–46% suppression). Mice fed a diet containing 1% aged garlic extract were partially protected from cis-urocanic acid-induced suppression of contact hypersensitivity, with greater protection from the lower concentrations of urocanic acid. Mice fed a diet containing 4% aged garlic extract were protected from all concentrations of urocanic acid. The results indicate that aged garlic extract contains ingredient(s) that **protect from UVB-induced suppression of contact hypersensitivity** and suggest that the mechanism of protection is **by antagonism of the cis-urocanic acid** mediation of this form of immunosuppression.

el-Mofty, M.M., Sakr, S.A. Essawy, A., Abdel Gawad, H.S. "Preventive action of garlic on aflatoxin B1-induced carcinogenesis in the toad Bufo regularis" *Nutr Cancer* (1994) 21(1):95–100

The action of **fresh minced garlic** and **garlic oil** on **aflatoxin B1**- (AFB1) induced **carcinogenesis** in the **toad** *Bufo regularis* was studied. Feeding toads with **AFB1 induced tumors in 19%** of the animals. Animals given AFB1 together with fresh garlic or garlic oil showed a **significant reduction in tumor incidence**. The tumor incidents were **3% and 9%** in animals given AFB1 plus garlic and AFB1 plus garlic oil, respectively. In all three groups, the tumors were located in the **liver (hepatocellular carcinomas)**, in addition to the **kidney** in animals treated with AFB1 alone and together with garlic. The kidney tumors were diagnosed as **metastatic** deposits from the primary liver tumors. It is speculated that one or more constituents of garlic may be responsible for inhibition of AFB1-induced carcinogenesis in B.

Gwilt, P.R., Lear, C.L., Tempero, M.A., Birt, D.D., Grandjean, A.C., Ruddon, R.W., Nagel, D.L. "The effect of garlic extract on human metabolism of acetaminophen" *Cancer Epidemiol Biomarkers Prev* (1994 Mar) 3(2):155–60

Several studies suggest that the constituents of garlic may inhibit experimentally induced carcinogenesis. To evaluate the **chemopreventive properties of garlic in humans**, the effects of chronic administration of an **aged garlic extract** on the disposition of **acetaminophen** and metabolites were studied. This commonly used drug was chosen because it **forms a reactive electrophilic metabolite after oxidative metabolism. Sixteen subjects** ingested **daily doses** of garlic extract (approximately equivalent to six to **seven cloves of garlic**) for **3 months**. Before the course of garlic, at the end of each month and 1 month after termination of garlic administration, a **1-g oral dose** of acetaminophen was given to each subject. **Plasma and urine** were measured for acetaminophen and the **glucuronide, sulfate, cysteinyl, mercapturate, and methylthio metabolites.** It was found that garlic treatment had **no discernible effect on oxidative metabolism** but was associated with a **slight increase in sulfate conjugation** of drug. These findings suggest that garlic extract has **limited potential as a chemopreventive agent.**

> Gwilt, P., Lear, C., Birt, D., Tempero, M., Grandjean, A., Ruddon, R., Nagel, D. "Modulation of human acetaminophen metabolism by garlic extract" (Meeting abstract) *Proc Annu Meet Am Assoc Cancer Res* (1993) 34:A3313 1993

The same authors repeated their study to evaluate the chemopreventive potential of garlic in humans and published their results in a different journal. This time the results were more encouraging. The effect of daily administration of an **aged garlic extract** (G) on **acetaminophen** (A) metabolism was studied in **18 healthy volunteers.** A was chosen as a model substrate because it is metabolized to an electrophilic intermediate which is conjugated by glutathione. Subjects ingested **10 ml of G daily for 3 mo.** Immediately prior to G treatment, at the end each month and one month after the G treatment, subjects ingested **1 gm of A** as 2 Tylenol caplets. Serial blood and urine samples were obtained and assayed for A, and the glucuronide, sulfate, 3-cysteinyl, 3-mercapturate and 3-methylthio metabolites using HPLC with tandem UV and electrochemical detection, pharmacokinetic analysis showed that the ingestion of G **increased formation of the sulfate and, to some extent, the glucuronide metabolites but had no effect on the oxidative metabolites.** Thus, one mechanism whereby garlic may act as a chemopreventive agent is by **shunting potential carcinogens away from activation pathways.**

Takada, N., Kitano, M,. Chen, T., Yano, Y., Otani, S., Fukushima, S. "Enhancing effects of organosulfur compounds from garlic and onions on hepatocarcinogenesis in rats: association with increased cell proliferation and elevated ornithine decarboxylase activity" *Jpn J Cancer Res* (1994 Nov) 85(11):1067–72

Four **organosulfur compounds** from garlic and onions were examined for modifying effects on *diethylnitrosamine (DEN)-induced neoplasia of the liver* in male F344 rats using the medium-term bioassay system based on the two-step model of hepatocarcinogenesis. Carcinogenic potential was scored by comparing the numbers and areas per cm^2 of induced glutathione S-transferase placental form-positive foci. **Isothiocyanic acid isobutyl ester (IAIE), dipropyl trisulfide (DPT),** and **allyl mercapton (AM)** exerted enhancing effects on their development, while **dimethyl trisulfide** also tended to increase them. To investigate possible mechanisms of the modifying influence, sequential changes in ornithine decarboxylase activity (ODC) over 24 h were measured in AM-treated liver tissue without prior DEN initiation. The activity started to increase by 4 h after AM-treatment, and reached maximum at 16 h, compared to controls. Spermidine/spermine N1-acetyltransferase activity was not significantly changed. An increase in proliferating cell nuclear antigen-positive cells followed the elevation of ODC activity. These results suggest that IAIE, DPT, and AM **promote rat hepatocarcinogenesis** and their promoting effect might be caused **by increased cell proliferation** with increased polyamine biosynthesis. *In evaluating relationships between diet and cancer, it is thus appropriate to consider not only a possible protective role of garlic and onions, but also enhancing effects.*

Matsuda, T., Takada, N., Yano, Y., Wanibuchi, H., Otani, S., Fukushima, S. "Dose-dependent inhibition of glutathione S-transferase placental form-positive hepatocellular foci induction in the rat by methyl propyl disulfide and propylene sulfide from garlic and onions" *Cancer Lett* (1994 Nov 11) 86(2):229–34

This article disputes the results of the previous reference. The same two organosulfur compounds, **methyl propyl disulfide (MPD)** and **propylene sulfide(PS)** from garlic and onions, were studied for their modifying effects on hepatocarcinogenesis in the F344 rats. Modifying potential was scored by comparing the number and area per cm^2 of induced glutathione S-transferase placental form (GST-P)-positive foci in the liver. MPD and PS significantly reduced both these parameters of GST-P-positive foci in a dose-dependent manner. To investigate possible mechanisms of inhibition, ornithine decarboxylase (ODC) and spermidine/spermine N1-acetyltransferase (SAT) activities were measured. In MPD and PS-high dose-treated liver tissue there was **tendency for their decrease, albeit non-significant, which suggested that the inhibitory effect** might have been **caused by decreased cell proliferation** associated with decreased polyamine biosynthesis. In evaluating relationships between diet and cancer, it is thus necessary to consider various effects in assessing possible protective roles of garlic and onions.

Ip, C., Lisk, D.J. "Enrichment of selenium in allium vegetables for cancer prevention" *Carcinogenesis* (1994 Sep) 15(9):1881–5

We previously reported that garlic cultivated with **selenium fertilization** is superior to regular garlic in **mammary cancer prevention** in the rat 7,12-dimethylbenz[a]anthracene (DMBA) model (Nutr. Cancer, 17, 279–286, 1992). A new crop of high-selenium garlic was harvested in 1992 and was used in a dose-response study to confirm the reproducibility of the product and the bioassay. **Supplementation of 1 or 2 p.p.m. Se in the diet** from the high-selenium garlic produced a **56% or 75% reduction respectively in the total tumor yield**. Since both garlic and onion belong to the same allium family of vegetables, we were also interested in finding out whether our experience with garlic could be similarly applied to onion. A high-selenium onion crop was grown in the same season and location and with the same schedule of selenium fertilization. Two distinct differences were noted with the **high-selenium onion** regarding its capacity to accumulate selenium and its efficacy in cancer prevention. First, the selenium *concentration* in onion was **considerably lower (28 p.p.m. Se dry wt)** as compared to that found in **garlic (110–150 p.p.m. Se)**. Second, given the same levels of selenium supplementation, the high-selenium onion was apparently not as powerful as the high-selenium garlic in mammary cancer inhibition. Thus different plants, even those of the same genus, may respond in their unique way to selenium fertilization and the biological benefits of selenium enrichment may vary depending on the species. Additional information from our study indicated that the high-selenium **garlic/onion might provide an ideal system for delivering selenium-substituted analogs in a food form for cancer prevention:**

(i) they expressed a good range of anticancer activity and could be easily adapted for human consumption on a regular basis;

(ii) their **ingestion did not result in an excessive accumulation of tissue selenium,** a concern that is associated with the standard selenium compounds such as **selenite** and **selenomethionine**;

(iii) no perturbation in the maintenance of functional selenoenzymes were observed even at high levels of supplementation.

Also presented at:

Ip, C., Lisk, D. "Potential of food modification in cancer prevention" (Meeting abstract) Anticarcinogenesis and Radiation Protection, 4th International Conference: Mechanisms, Biomarkers, Molecular Diagnostics and Preventive Strategies. April 18–23, 1993, Baltimore, Maryland, 1993. :48

Amagase, H., Milner, J.A. "Impact of dietary lipids on the ability of garlic to inhibit 7,12-dimethylbenz(a)anthracene (DMBA) binding to mammary DNA (Meeting abstract) *FASEB J* (1993) 7(3):A69 1993

Female SD rats were fed the experimental diet for 2 wk prior to DMBA treatment (25 mg/kg body wt). DMBA-DNA adducts were quantitated using a 32P-postlabeling technique. In experiment 1, rats were **fed diets with or without 2% garlic** and varying amounts of **corn oil (5, 10 or 20%)**. **Increasing dietary corn oil** resulted in a proportional **increase in DMBA-DNA binding**. The depression in total and individual DMBA-DNA adducts resulting from garlic consumption was greatest in rats fed 20% corn oil.

Experiment 2 examined the influence of source of lipid (**15% corn, olive, coconut or fish oil**) added to basal diets containing 5% corn oil. Regardless of source, consumption of diets containing 20% lipid increased DMBA-DNA binding by approx 100% compared to diets containing 5% dietary corn oil. **Garlic depressed DMBA-DNA binding by 50, 29 and 70% when diets contained 20% corn, olive or fish oil, respectively**. Although **coconut oil** increased the formation of DMBA-DNA adducts, **garlic failed** to reduce the binding when this source of lipid was provided. These studies demonstrate an effect of several sources of **lipids on the initiation phase of carcinogenesis**. Furthermore, these studies suggest the effect of

garlic is dependent upon the degree of unsaturation of the dietary lipid fed.

Ip, C., Lisk, D.J. "Bioavailability of selenium from selenium-enriched garlic" *Nutr Cancer* (1993) 20(2):129–37

We previously reported that garlic grown in a selenium-fertilized medium (selenium-enriched garlic) is superior to regular garlic in mammary cancer prevention in an animal model (Nutr Cancer 17, 279–286, 1992). The present study was designed to evaluate the nutritional bioavailability of selenium from this garlic with use of two liver selenoenzymes as biomarkers: **glutathione peroxidase** and **type I 5'-deiodinase. Rats** were **fed a selenium-deficient diet** (0.01ppm Se) from **weaning for four weeks** to deplete both enzymes. They were **then supplemented** with nutritional levels of **selenium (0.1–0.5 ppm)** in the form of **sodium selenite** (positive control) or **selenium-enriched garlic.** Our results showed that selenium-enriched garlic was just as effective as selenite in restoring the activity of both selenoenzymes. This was demonstrated in a time course repletion experiment as well as in a dose-response experiment. Thus the **selenium in selenium-enriched garlic has potent nutritional and anticancer efficacy.** The type I 5'-deiodinase enzyme catalyzes the conversion of thyroxine (T4) to 3,5,3'-triiodothyronine (T3) and is responsible for most of the circulating T3. Because cancer chemoprevention by selenium usually requires pharmacological levels of selenium, we also examined the possible modulation of type I 5'-deiodinase by long-term feeding of selenium-enriched garlic at 3 ppm Se in the diet. The observation that a high intake of selenium-enriched garlic did not affect 5'-deiodinase activity suggests that its anticarcinogenic effect is unlikely to be mediated by an imbalance in the blood T4-to-T3 ratio.

Morioka, N., Sze, L.L. Morton, D.L., Irie, R.F. "A protein fraction from aged garlic extract enhances cytotoxicity and proliferation of human lymphocytes mediated by interleukin-2 and concanavalin A" *Cancer Immunol Immunother* (1993 Oct) 37(5):316–22

Fraction 4 (F4), a protein fraction isolated from aged garlic extract, enhanced cytotoxicity of human peripheral blood lymphocytes (PBL) against both natural-killer (NK)-sensitive K562 and NK-resistant M14 cell lines. Although F4 treatment alone increased cytotoxicity, the effect was **more remarkable** when F4 was administered **together with suboptimal doses of interleukin-2** (IL-2); combination treatment of **5 micrograms/ml** F4 **plus 10 U/ml IL-2** for 72 h generated lymphokine-activated killer activity **equivalent to** that produced by **100 U/ml IL-2 alone** against M14. F4 enhanced IL-2-induced proliferation and IL-2 receptor (Tac) expression of PBL without significant increase of IL-2 production. The enhancement of cytotoxicity both by F4 alone and by F4 plus IL-2 was abolished by anti-IL-2 antibody. F4 also **enhanced concanavalin-A(ConA)-induced proliferation of PBL**. Radiolabeled-ConA binding assays revealed that F4 treatment **greatly augmented the affinity** and **slightly increased the number of ConA binding sites in PBL**. F4 also enhanced ConA-induced IL-2 receptor (Tac) expression and IL-2 production of PBL. Anti- IL-2 antibody inhibited the effect of F4 on ConA-induced proliferation. These data suggest that IL-2 is involved in the augmentative effects of F4. Our results indicate that **F4 is a very efficient immunopotentiator and may be used for immunotherapy**.

El-Bayoumy, K., Ip, C., Chae, Y.H., Upadhyaya, P., Lisk, D., Prokopczyk, B. "Mammary cancer chemoprevention by diallyl selenide, a novel organoselenium compound"

(Meeting abstract) *Proc Annu Meet Am Assoc Cancer Res* (1993) 34:A3322 1993

Extensive ongoing studies indicate that **organoselenium compounds** are **superior to their sulfur analogs** as **chemopreventive agents**. Plants are known to convert inorganic selenite to organoselenium analogs of naturally occurring sulfur compounds. It has been reported previously that garlic cultivated in a selenium-fertilized medium has a greater anticarcinogenic activity than regular garlic (Nutr Cancer 17:279, 1992). The above findings suggest that the incorporation of selenium into garlic, which contains an abundant source of a variety of allyl sulfides, may enhance its potential attributes in cancer protection. A possible candidate in selenium-enriched garlic is **diallyl selenide (DASe)**. The latter was **synthesized** and was found to be **about 300x more active than diallyl sulfide** in **inhibiting rat mammary tumor** development induced by 7,12-dimethylbenz[a]anthracene (DMBA). DASe **also** inhibited DMBA-DNA adduct formation in the **liver**.

Hatono, S., Velasco, M.A., Palmer, C., Wargovich, M.J. "Chemopreventive activity of sulfur-containing compounds derived from garlic" (Meeting abstract) *Proc Annu Meet Am Assoc Cancer Res* (1993) 34:A744 1993

In this study, chemopreventive activity of sulfur-containing compounds were determined using **azoxymethane (AOM)-induced colonic aberrant crypt assay**. Sprague-Dawley **rats** (7 wk old) were fed the purified diet (AIN-76A) during the acclimation (1 wk) and experiment (4 wk). **50 mg/kg of S-allyl cysteine (SAC)** was administered **po 15 min and 3 hr prior to two weekly ip AOM injections (15 mg/kg)**. **Three weeks after the last AOM injection**, the colon was removed and stained with methylene blue. **100 to 200 aberrant crypts per rat** were found in the control group (av 145 +/- 7.4). In both SAC-treated groups, the development of **aberrant crypts was significantly reduced 64.0%** (p less than 0.05). Additionally, SAC **significantly increased the glutathione-S-transferase activity in the liver.** These results suggest that the compounds are **potentially anticarcinogenic, possibly by enhancing metabolic detoxification of carcinogen.**

Radical Scavenging Antioxidant

Yamasaki, T., Li, L., Lau, B.H. "Garlic extract protects vascular endothelial cells from oxidant injury" (Meeting abstract) *Proc Annu Meet Am Assoc Cancer Res* (1993) 34:A3299 1993

Oxygen radical injury and **lipid peroxidation** have been suggested as major causes of cancer, atherosclerosis and the aging process. In this study, we examined in vitro the effect of garlic on H_2O_2-**induced oxidant injury in bovine pulmonary artery endothelial cells (PAEC).** After overnight preincubation with aged garlic extract (AGE, from Wakunaga Pharmaceutical Co, Ltd, Japan), PAEC monolayers were exposed to H_2O_2 for 3 hr. Cell viability (MTT assay), lactate dehydrogenase (LDH) release, and lipid peroxidation (malondialdehyde; MDA) were measured to assess oxidant injury. AGE (1–2 mg/ml) **pretreatment significantly reduced the loss of cell viability** induced by 25–100 uM of H_2O_2. AGE also exhibited **dose-dependent inhibition of both LDH release and MDA production** induced by 50 uM of H_2O_2. The results show that AGE can **protect vascular endothelial cells from oxidant injury.** These data suggest that AGE contains certain radical scavengers, and may thus be **useful for prevention of cancer, atherosclerosis, and for retardation of the aging process.**

Imai, J., Ide, N., Nagae, S., Moriguchi, T., Matsuura, H., Itakura, Y. "Antioxidant and radical scavenging effects of aged garlic extract and its constituents" *Planta Med* (1994 Oct) 60(5):417–20

The antioxidant properties of three garlic preparations and organosulfur compounds in garlic have been determined. **Aged garlic extract** *inhibited the emission of low level chemiluminescence and the early formation of thiobarbituric acid-reactive substances (TBA-RS) in liver microsomal fraction initiated by t-butyl hydroperoxide.* However, the **water extracts of raw and heat-treated garlic** enhanced the emission of low level chemiluminescence. Among the variety of organosulfur compounds, **S-allylcysteine (SAC)** and **S-allylmercaptocysteine (SAMC),** the major organosulfur compounds found in aged garlic extract, showed **radical scavenging activity** in both chemiluminescence and 1,1-diphenyl-2-picrylhydrazyl (DPPH) assays, indicating that these compounds may play an important role in the antioxidative activity of aged garlic extract.

Torok, B., Belagyi, J., Rietz, B., Jacob, R. "Effectiveness of garlic on the radical activity in radical generating systems" *Arzneimittelforschung* (1994 May) 44(5):608–11

The **radical scavenging capacity** of garlic (allium sativum) has been investigated **in vitro** in radical generating systems by **electron paramagnetic resonance (EPR) and low-level chemiluminescence** measurements. Garlic (both the homogenate of 10% in physiological saline solution and its supernatant) was able to reduce the radicals generated by the Fenton reaction and trapped by phenyl-butyl-nitron for EPR measurements. Also radicals present in **cigarette smoke** could be reduced by garlic as judged from chemiluminescence in the presence of tert.-butyl-hydroperoxide. According to the in vitro measurements garlic contains substances which have significant radical scavenging capacity.

Lewin, G., Popov, I. "Antioxidant effects of aqueous garlic extract. 2nd communication: Inhibition of the Cu(2+)-initiated oxidation of low density lipoproteins" *Arzneimittelforschung* (1994 May) 44(5):604–7

The **aqueous extract** from the garlic preparation **Kwai** the antioxidant effect of which has been previously detected by the authors using the method of photochemiluminescence was tested in respect of the **Cu(2+)-initiated oxidation of low density lipoprotein (LDL)**. The formation of conjugated diene which accompanies the lipid peroxidation process was detected photometrically. In this test system too, a **dose-related oxidation-inhibiting effect** of the extract was established. Further experiments will be required to find out whether such effect is due to the reduction of intrinsic antioxidants or to the increase of the integral antioxidant capacity of LDL.

Popov, I., Blumstein, A., Lewin, G. "Antioxidant effects of aqueous garlic extract. 1st communication: Direct detection using the photochemiluminescence" *Arzneimittelforschung* (1994 May) 44(5):602–4

The antioxidant effect of the **aqueous extract** from the garlic preparation **Kwai** was investigated using the method of **photochemiluminescence**. The method is based on the photo-induced, **superoxide radical mediated autoxidation of luminol**, and allows for the capability of substances to inhibit the free radical processes in this test system to be quantified, and hence for their antioxidant properties in respect of a standard substance (e.g. ascorbic acid, alpha-tocopherol) to be compared. The aqueous extract obtained from **1mg of the garlic preparation** was found to be **anti-oxidatively as effective as 30 nmol of ascorbic acid** and/or **3.6 nmol of alpha-tocopherol**.

Antiplatelet Antithrombotic

Kiesewetter, H., Jung, F., Jung, E.M., Blume, J., Mrowietz, C., Birk, A., Koscielny, J., Wenzel, E. "Effects of garlic coated tablets in peripheral arterial occlusive disease" *Clin Investig* (1993 May) 71(5):383–6

For the first time, a weak clinical efficacy of a **12-week therapy** with **garlic powder (daily dose, 800 mg)** is demonstrated in patients with **peripheral arterial occlusive disease stage II**. The **increase in walking distance** in the verum group **by 46 m** (from 161.0 +/- 65.1 to 207.1 +/- 85.0 m) was significantly higher (P 0.05) than in the **placebo group (by 31 m**, from 172.0 +/- 60.9 to 203.1 +/- 72.8). **Both groups received physical therapy twice a week**. The diastolic blood pressure, spontaneous thrombocyte aggregation, plasma viscosity, and cholesterol concentration also decreased significantly. Body weight was maintained. It is quite interesting that the **garlic-specific increase in walking distance** did **not appear to occur until the 5th week of treatment,** connected **with a simultaneous decrease in spontaneous thrombocyte aggregation**. Therefore, garlic may be an appropriate agent especially for the long-term treatment of an **incipient intermittent claudication**.

Mutsch-Eckner, M., Erdelmeier, C.A., Sticher, O., Reuter, H.D. "A novel amino acid glycoside and three amino acids from Allium sativum" *J Nat Prod* (1993 Jun) 56(6):864–9

A novel **amino acid glycoside (-)-N-(1'-deoxy-1'-beta-D- fructopyranosyl)-S-allyl-L-cysteine sulfoxide [1], was isolated from a hydrophilic extract of the leaves** of Allium sativum (Alliaceae), together with three known compounds: (+)-S-allyl-L-cysteine sulfoxide [2],(+)-S-methyl-L-cysteine sulfoxide [3], and (+)-S-(trans-1-propenyl)-L-cysteine sulfoxide [4]. The latter two substances were isolated for the first time from garlic. The structure elucidation of 1 was performed by extensive chemical, spectroscopic (ir, fabms, 1D and 2D(1)H- and (13)C-nmr measurements) and chromatographic experiments. For the first time, detailed nmr data and the unambiguous assignment of all (13)C-nmr data for compounds 2–4 were reported. Compound 1, the amino acid glycoside, **revealed a inhibition of in vitro platelet aggregation induced by ADP and epinephrine**, whereas none of the amino acids tested displayed any activity.

Apitz-Castro, R., Badimon, J.J., Badimon, L. "A garlic derivative, ajoene, inhibits platelet deposition on severely damaged vessel wall in an in vivo porcine experimental model" *Thromb Res* (1994 Aug 1) 75(3):243–9

Ajoene, (E,Z)-4,5,9-trithiadodeca-1,6,11-triene 9-oxide, is a potent **antiplatelet** compound isolated from alcoholic extracts of garlic. In vitro, ajoene **reversibly inhibits platelet aggregation** as well as the release reaction induced by all known agonists. We used a well characterized perfusion chamber to study the **in vivo** effects of ajoene on *platelet deposition onto a highly thrombogenic, severely damaged arterial wall, obtained by stripping off the intimal layer and exposing tunica media.* Platelet-vessel wall interaction and the effect of ajoene was studied under flow conditions of high and low local shear rate that mimic laminar blood flow in small and medium size arteries (1690 sec-1 and 212 sec-1). Our results indicate that **administration of ajoene to heparinized animals, significantly prevents thrombus formation at local low blood shear rate.** Ajoene does not inhibit binding of vWF to GPIb, therefore, **it does not affect platelet adhesion.** In fact, although ajoene **impairs fibrinogen** and vWF (less efficient) binding to GPIIb/IIIa, it **does not totally inhibits platelet deposition** to the substrates at any of the shear rates used in this study. Our present results, under in vivo flow conditions and in the presence of physiological calcium levels, suggest that *ajoene may be potentially useful for the acute prevention of thrombus formation* induced by severe vascular damage, mainly in arterial sites with local low shear rates.

Kiesewetter, H., Jung, F., Jung, E.M., Mroweitz, C., Koscielny, J., Wenzel, E. "Effect of garlic on platelet aggregation in patients with increased risk of juvenile ischaemic attack" *Eur J Clin Pharmacol* (1993) 45(4):333–6

A **platelet-inhibiting effect** is described for garlic. In this double-blind, placebo-controlled study on **60 voluntary subjects** with cerebrovascular risk factors and constantly increased platelet aggregation it was demonstrated that the **daily ingestion of 800 mg of powdered garlic** (in the form of coated tablets) **over 4 weeks** led to a **significant inhibition** of the pathologically increased **ratio of circulating platelet aggregates and of spontaneous platelet aggregation. The ratio of circulating platelet aggregates decreased by 10.3%**, from 1.17 +/- 0.08 to 1.05 +/- 0.11 (P 0.01), and spontaneous platelet aggregation by **56.3%**, from 40.7 +/- 23.3 to 17.8 +/- 23.2 degrees (P 0.01) during the garlic phase. There were no significant changes in the placebo group. The parallel group comparison (garlic versus placebo) revealed a significantly different ratio of circulating platelet aggregates after 4 weeks of treatment (P 0.05). After the **4-week wash-out phase** the values increased again to 1.19 +/- 0.32 and 34.9 +/- 28.7 degrees, reaching the initial values (run-in phase prior to the ingestion of garlic). Since garlic is well tolerated it would be worth testing it in a controlled clinical trial for usefulness in preventing disease manifestations associated with platelet aggregation.

Antiarrhythmic

Isensee, H., Rietz, B., Jacob, R. "Cardioprotective actions of garlic (Allium sativum)" *Arzneimittelforschung* (1993 Feb) 43(2):94–8

The influence of an intake of **garlic powder** (1%— corresponding to Kwai/Sapec—added to a standard chow for a **10-week** period) on the **susceptibility to ventricular arrhythmias under ischemia** and reperfusion was investigated in the **isolated rat heart** (Langendorff preparation) perfused with a modified Krebs-Henseleit solution. The **incidence of ventricular tachycardia (VT) and fibrillation (VF) after ligation** of the descending branch of the left coronary artery **(LAD) (20 min)** was **significantly reduced in the garlic group** as compared to untreated controls **(VT: 0% vs. 35.5%; VF: 50% vs. 88%)**. The **size of the ischemic zone was significantly smaller (31.7% vs. 40.9%** of total heart tissue). The **reperfusion** experiments **(5 min after 10 min ischemia)** revealed similar results **(VT: 50% vs. 100%; VF: 30% vs. 90%)**. The **time until occurrence of extrasystoles and VT or VF was prolonged** in most cases, and the **duration of arrhythmias was abbreviated. No significant alterations in cardiac membrane fatty acid composition could be found.** The significance of free radical scavenging activity of garlic for its antiarrhythmic effects has to be established.

Rietz, B., Isensee, H., Strobach, H., Makdessi, S., Jacob, R. "Cardioprotective actions of wild garlic (allium ursinum) in ischemia and reperfusion" *Mol Cell Biochem* (1993 Feb 17) 119(1–2):143–50

The **susceptibility to ventricular arrhythmias** under the conditions of cardiac ischemia and reperfusion was investigated in the Langendorff heart preparation of rats fed for eight weeks a standard chow enriched with **2% of**

pulverized wild garlic leaves. The isolated hearts were perfused with a modified Krebs-Henseleit solution. The incidence of **ventricular fibrillation (VF) during 20 min occlusion** of the descending branch of the left coronary artery **(LAD)** was **significantly reduced** in the wild garlic group as compared to untreated controls **(20% vs 88%).** The same holds for the **size of the ischemic zone (33.6% vs 40.9%** of heart weight). In the **reperfusion** experiments (5 min after 10 min ischemia), **ventricular tachycardia (VT) occurred in 70%** of the wild garlic group vs 100% in untreated controls and **VF in 50% vs 90%.** The **time until occurrence of extrasystoles, VT or VR was prolonged.** No significant alterations in cardiac fatty acid composition could be observed.

Although the prostacyclin production was slightly increased in hearts of the wild garlic group, inhibition of cyclooxygenase by acetylsalicylic acid (ASA; aspirin) could not completely prevent the cardioprotective effects suggesting that the prostaglandin system does not play a decisive role in the cardioprotective action of wild garlic. Furthermore, a **moderate angiotensin converting enzyme (ACE) inhibiting action** of wild garlic was found in vitro as well as in vivo that could **contribute to the cardioprotective and blood pressure lowering action** of wild garlic. Whether a free radical scavenging activity of wild garlic is involved in its cardioprotective effects remains to be established.

Martin, N., Bardisa, L., Pantoja, C., Vargas, M., Quezada, P., Valenzuela, J. "Anti-arrhythmic profile of a garlic dialysate assayed in dogs and isolated atrial preparations" *J Ethnopharmacol* (1994 Jun) 43(1):1–8

The effects of garlic (Allium sativum L., Liliaceae) dialysate were studied on **arrhythmias** induced in **anaesthetized dogs** and on **isolated left rat atria**. Garlic dialysate **suppressed premature ventricular contractions (PVC)** and **ventricular tachycardia (VT)** in **ouabain-in-toxicated dogs** as well as the ectopic rhythms induced by **isoprenaline** (10(-6) M) and **aconitine** (10(-8) M) on **electrically driven left rat atria**. The **effective refractory period (ERP)** and the **sinus node recovery time (SNRT)** of isolated rat atria were **prolonged** in a **dose-dependent** manner by the administration of this extract. **Garlic dialysate** decreased the positive inotropic and chronotropic effects of isoprenaline in a concentration-dependent manner. These last effects were increased by propranolol. The results suggest that garlic dialysate has a **significant antiarrhythmic effect in both ventricular and supraventricular arrhythmias.**

Pharmakokinetics and Distribution

Lachmann, G., Lorenz, D., Radeck, W., Steiper, M.
"[The pharmacokinetics of the 35S labeled labeled garlic constituents alliin, allicin and vinyldithiine]
Untersuchungen zur Pharmakokinetik der mit 35S markierten Knoblauchinhaltsstoffe Alliin, Allicin und Vinyldithiine" *Arzneimittelforschung* (1994 Jun) 44(6):734–43

Three groups of 3 **rats** received oral doses (8 mg/kg) of garlic constituents (**alliin, allicin and vinyldithiines (2-vinyl-[4H]-1,3- dithiine and 3-vinyl-[4H]-1,2-dithiine))** in the form of an oil macerate of the 35S-labeled substance. The measured activity was referred to 35S-alliin (35S-alliin equivalents). The blood activity levels in each group were monitored for 72 h. For 35S-allicin and the labeled vinyldithiines the **excretion** with the **urine, feces, and exhaled air** was also measured. The distribution among the organs (whole-body autoradiography) and the urinary metabolite pattern (thin-layer chromatography) were also determined. For 35S-alliin the blood activity profile differed considerably from those of 35S-allicin and the labeled vinyldithiines: both the absorption and the elimination of the radioactivity were distinctly faster than for the other garlic constituents, **maximum blood levels being reached within the first 10 min** and elimination from the blood being almost complete after 6 h. For the other garlic constituents the maximum blood levels were not reached until 30–60 min (35S-allicin) or 120 min (vinyldithiines) p.a. and blood levels 1000 ng-Eq/ml were still present at the end of the study after 72 h. The mean total urinary and fecal excretion after 72 h was 85.5% (35S-allicin) or 92.3% (labeled vinyldithiines) of the dose. The urinary excretion indicates a minimum absorption rate of 65% (35S-allicin) or 73% (vinyldithiines). It is uncertain whether the 19–21% recovered in the feces was unabsorbed substance or had been excreted via the bile or intestinal mucosa. The exhaled air showed only traces of activity although the **whole-body autoradiographs**, after fairly long exposure (96 h), **showed distinct enrichment of activity in the mucosa of the airways and pharynx**. The activity is **deposited** mainly in the cartilage of the **vertebral column and ribs**. There was no detectable difference in organ distribution between 35S-allicin and the labeled vinyldithiines. All that could be established from the urinary metabolite pattern was that unchanged 35S-allicin and unchanged labeled vinyldithiines are absent. There is therefore **extensive metabolization**. The **metabolites must have a very polar structure with acid functional groups** since satisfactory separation was achievable only with acid solvent systems. Conjugates with sulfuric or glucuronic acid were not detectable. These results reveal no differences in pharmacokinetic behavior between 35S-allicin and the labeled vinyldithiines. A final verdict as to whether the metabolites, which may be pharmacologically active, are identical must await further studies designed to identify the metabolites.

Antiatherogenic Lipid Reduction

Gebhardt, R. "Multiple inhibitory effects of garlic extracts on cholesterol biosynthesis in hepatocytes" *Lipids* (1993 Jul) 28(7):613–9

Exposure of **primary rat hepatocytes** and **human HepG2 cells** to **water-soluble garlic extracts** resulted in the concentration-dependent **inhibition of cholesterol biosynthesis** at several different enzymatic steps. At low concentrations, **sterol biosynthesis** from [14C]acetate was **decreased in rat** hepatocytes by **23%** with an IC50 (half-maximal inhibition) value of 90 micrograms/mL and **in HepG2 cells by 28%** with an IC50 value of 35 micrograms/mL. This inhibition was exerted **at the** level of **hydroxymethylglutaryl-CoA reductase (HMG-CoA reductase)** as indicated by direct enzymatic measurements and the absence of inhibition if [14C]mevalonate was used as a precursor. **At high concentrations (above 0.5 mg/mL), inhibition** of cholesterol biosynthesis was not only **seen** at an early step where it increased considerably with dose, but **also at later steps** resulting in the accumulation of the precursors lanosterol and 7-dehydrocholesterol. No desmosterol was formed which, however, was a major precursor accumulating in the presence of triparanol. Thus, the accumulation of sterol precursors seems to be of less therapeutic significance during consumption of garlic, because it requires concentrations one or two orders of magnitude above those affecting HMG-CoA reductase. **Alliin**, the main sulfur-containing compound of garlic, was **without effect** itself. If converted to **allicin**, it resulted in similar changes of the sterol pattern. This suggested that the latter compound **might contribute**

to the inhibition at the late steps. In contrast, **nicotinic acid** and particularly **adenosine** caused moderate inhibition of HMG-CoA reductase activity and of cholesterol biosynthesis suggesting that these compounds participate, at least in part, in the early inhibition of sterol synthesis by garlic extracts.

Kenzelmann, R., Kade, F. "Limitation of the deterioration of lipid parameters by a standardized garlic-ginkgo combination product. A multicenter placebo-controlled double-blind study" *Arzneimittelforschung* (1993 Sep) 43(9):978–81

The efficacy of a **garlic-ginkgo combination product (Allium plus)** was analyzed in a randomized placebo-controlled double-blind study under extreme dietary conditions. The **Christmas/New Year's season** was chosen for this **2 months** lasting investigation analyzing whether the known cholesterol lowering effect of garlic was even effective during the period of the year with the most cholesterol-rich meals. **43 patients** with **elevated total cholesterol** levels ranging between **230–390 mg/dl** completed the study. There were **no significant changes** of the **total cholesterol values in both treatment groups.** Nevertheless the analysis of improvement or deterioration of total cholesterol values revealed **a clear difference between verum and placebo. 20%** of the patients in the **placebo** group showed an **improvement** of their total cholesterol level, while there was a significant greater improvement rate of **35% in the verum group** (p 0.05). The **responders** of the verum group showed a **reduction** in the **total cholesterol** values from 298.5 +/- 53.8 to 293.0 +/- 56.4 mg/dl after 1 month and a total reduction of **10.4% after 2 months** to 267.6 +/- 44.4 mg/dl. The difference after 2 months of treatment was significantly different from the starting value (p 0.05). After the 2 months treatment phase there was a **2 weeks wash-out period.** During this period the **total cholesterol value returned to 293.5 +/-** 90.1 mg/dl showing the effectiveness of garlic treatment, but **indicating the need for a continuous long-term therapy**.

> Heinle, H., Betz, E. "Effects of dietary garlic supplementation in a rat model of atherosclerosis" *Arzneimittelforschung* (1994 May) 44(5):614–7

In the present study possible **antiatherogenic effects** of dietary garlic were investigated in an experimental model which consists in the **deendothelialisation by ballooning** of the **a. carotis communis of rats**. 3 experimental groups were established: group I received a **standard diet**; the diet of group II was supplemented with **2% cholesterol** and group III received **2% cholesterol and 5% dried garlic powder**. **Four weeks** after ballooning **plasma cholesterol**, the **average thickness of the neointima** as well as the **DNA content** and the expression of **collagens type I, III and IV** in the ballooned arterial segment were determined. Furthermore, the specific activities of the enzymes **glutathione peroxidase, glutathione disulfide reductase, glutathione-S-transferase and glucose 6 phosphate dehydrogenase** were measured in homogenates of liver, heart and aorta. Hypercholesterolemia induced by cholesterol-feeding (group II 92 +/- 18 mg/100 ml) was **significantly reduced by garlic** (group III 53 +/- 19 mg/100 ml). Only little effects of garlic were seen in inhibiting neointima after ballooning. However, **significant** effects were found in **protecting** the **enzymes of the glutathione dependent peroxide detoxification system,** which is **strongly impaired under hypercholesterolemia**. Generally a normalisation, in some cases even an improvement beyond that, of the enzyme activities occurred in the garlic treated group. This indicates that in the model of atherosclerosis used here **garlic is effective in lowering plasma choles-**

terol and in **improving peroxide detoxification**, however, it has only **little influence on the wound healing** reaction and does **not significantly inhibit the development of intimal thickenings** after ballooning.

Yeh, Y.Y., Yeh, S.M. "Garlic reduces plasma lipids by inhibiting hepatic cholesterol and triacylglycerol synthesis" *Lipids* (1994 Mar) 29(3):189–93

Prompted by the reported **hypolipidemic activity** of garlic, the present study was undertaken to elucidate the mechanism(s) underlying the cholesterol-lowering effects of garlic. **Rat hepatocytes in primary culture** were used to determine the short-term effects of garlic preparations on [1-14C]acetate and [2-3H]glycerol incorporation into cholesterol, fatty acids and glycerol lipids. When compared with the control group, cells treated with a high concentration of garlic extracts [i.e., petroleum ether- (PEF), methanol- (MEF) and water-extractable (WEF) fractions from fresh garlic] showed **decreased rates of [1-14C]acetate incorporation into cholesterol (by 37–64%) and into fatty acids (by 28–64%). Kyolic** containing S-allyl cysteine and organosulfur compounds inhibited cholesterogenesis in a concentration dependent manner with a **maximum inhibition of 87%** at 0.4 mM. At this concentration, Kyolic decreased [1-14C]acetate incorporation into fatty acids by 67%. S-allyl cysteine at 2.0 and 4.0 mM inhibited cholesterogenesis by 20–25%. PEF, MEF and WEF depressed the rates of [2-3H]glycerol incorporation into triacylglycerol, diacylglycerol and phospholipids in the presence of acetate, but not in the presence of oleate. The results suggest that the **hypocholesterolemic effect** of garlic stems, in part, from **decreased hepatic cholesterogenesis**, whereas the **triacylglycerol-lowering** effect appears to be due to **inhibition of fatty acid synthesis.**

Silagy, C., Neil, A. "Garlic as a lipid lowering agent—a meta-analysis" *J R Coll Physicians Lond* (1994 Jan-Feb) 28(1):39–45

Garlic supplements may have an important role to play in the treatment of **hypercholesterolaemia**. To determine the effect of garlic on serum lipids and lipoproteins relative to placebo and other lipid lowering agents, a systematic review, including meta-analysis, was undertaken of published and unpublished randomised controlled trials of garlic preparations of at least four weeks' duration.

Sixteen trials, with data from **952 subjects**, were included in the analyses. The pooled mean difference in the absolute change (from baseline to final measurement in mmol/l) of total serum cholesterol, triglycerides, and high-density lipoprotein (HDL)-cholesterol was compared between subjects treated with garlic therapy against those treated with placebo or other agents. The mean difference in reduction of total cholesterol between garlic-treated subjects and those receiving placebo (or avoiding garlic in their diet) was -0.77 mmol/l (95% CI: -0.65, -0.89 mmol/l). These changes represent a **12% reduction with garlic therapy** beyond the final levels achieved with placebo alone. The reduction was evident **after one month of therapy and persisted for at least six months**. In the dried garlic powders, in which the allicin content is standardized, there was **no significant difference in the size of the reduction across the dose range of 600–900 mg daily**. Dried garlic powder preparations also significantly lowered serum triglyceride by 0.31 mmol/l compared to placebo (95% CI: -0.14, -0.49).

Phelps, S., Harris, W.S. "Garlic supplementation and lipoprotein oxidation susceptibility" *Lipids* (1993 May) 28(5):475–7

Ten healthy volunteers were given **600 mg/d of garlic powder (6 tablets of Kwai) for two weeks** in a placebo-controlled, randomized, double-blind crossover trial. We found that although **serum lipid and lipoprotein levels were not lowered in this short time period**, the ex vivo **susceptibility of apolipoprotein B-containing lipoproteins to oxidation was significantly decreased (-34%)**. Because garlic has been reported to beneficially affect serum lipid levels, platelet function, fibrinolysis and blood pressure, this **additional effect of retarding lipoprotein oxidation** may contribute to the **potential antiatherosclerotic effect** of garlic.

Heavy Metal Detoxification

Hanafy, M.S., Shalaby, S.M., el-Fouly, M.A. Abd el-Aziz, M.I., Soliman, F.A. "Effect of garlic on lead contents in chicken tissues" *DTW Dtsch Tierarztl Wochenschr* (1994 Apr) 101(4):157–8

Lead has been implicated in the etiology of human and animal diseases. In view of earlier literature indicating that garlic antagonized lead toxicity, we have investigated the possible use of garlic feeding to clean up lead contents from **chickens** which had been exposed to **natural or experimental lead pollution** and consequently eliminate one of the sources of lead pollution to human consumers. Groups of chickens (10 birds each) were given lead alone (lead acetate equivalent to 5 mg lead/kg B.W.) or both lead and garlic simultaneously or lead followed by garlic post-treatment or garlic alone or distilled water. **Lead concentrations were reduced** in **muscle and liver tissues** of chickens given both lead and garlic simultaneously or as a post-treatment. Reduction in tissue-lead concentrations were **greater** in birds given garlic **as a post-treatment than** those given garlic **simultaneously with lead.** The results indicate that **garlic contains chelating compounds** capable of enhancing elimination of lead. Garlic feeding can be exploited to safeguard human consumers by minimizing lead concentrations in meat of food animals which had been grown in a lead polluted environment.

Neonatal Nursing Behavior

Mennella, J.A., Beauchamp, G.K. "The effects of repeated exposure to garlic-flavored milk on the nursling's behavior" *Pediatr Res* (1993 Dec) 34(6):805–8

The present study investigated whether prior **consumption of garlic** by **nursing mothers** modifies their **infant's behaviors during breast-feeding** when the mothers again consume garlic. Three groups of mother-infant dyads were studied. The groups differed in the type (placebo or garlic) or the timing (d 5–7 or 8–10) of capsule ingestion by the mothers and, consequently, in the amount and recency of exposure their infants had to garlic-flavored milk during an 11-day experimental period. Each mother-infant pair was observed during two 4-h test sessions. The first session occurred at the beginning of the experimental period, when the mothers ingested placebo capsules (day 4); the second occurred at the end of the experimental period, when they ingested garlic capsules (day 11). During test sessions, the infants fed on demand and were weighed before and after each breast-feeding to determine the amount of milk ingested, and their behaviors during breast-feeding were monitored by videotape. The results demonstrated an effect of prior experience with garlic in mother's milk. The infants who had no exposure to garlic volatiles in their mothers' milk during the experimental period spent significantly more **time breast-feeding after their mothers ingested garlic** capsules compared with those infants whose mothers repeatedly consumed garlic during the experimental period. Moreover, the former group of **infants spent significantly more time attached to their mothers' breasts** during the 4-h test session in which their mothers ingested the garlic compared with the session in which she ingested the placebo.

Anti-inflammatory

Ali, M., Angelo-Khattar, M., Farid, A., Hassan, R.A., Thulesius, O. "Aqueous extracts of garlic (Allium sativum) inhibit prostaglandin synthesis in the ovine ureter" *Prostaglandins Leukot Essent Fatty Acids* (1993 Nov) 49(5):855–9

The **prostaglandins** (PGs) synthesized **from C14-arachidonic acid** by the homogenized **sheep ureter** were identified as being prostacyclin (PGI2), PGF2 alpha and thromboxane B2 (TXB2). The **radioimmunoassay** (RIA) estimation of 6-keto-PGF1 alpha, a stable metabolite of PGI2, confirms that it was the major metabolite of arachidonic acid. **Aqueous extracts of fresh garlic (5, 12.5, 25 and 50 mg/ml)** were shown to **inhibit the synthesis of the prostanoids in a dose dependent manner. Fresh garlic extracts (1, 2.5, 5 and 10 mg/ml)** also dose dependently **inhibited spontaneous rhythmic contractions** of the isolated ureter. **Boiled garlic** (5, 12.5, 25 and 50 mg/ml) had **no effect** on either ureteral motility or the PG synthesizing capacity of the sheep ureter.